EVALUATION
DESIGN
FOR COMPLEX
GLOBAL
INITIATIVES

WORKSHOP SUMMARY

Steve Olson, *Rapporteur*

Board on Global Health

INSTITUTE OF MEDICINE
OF THE NATIONAL ACADEMIES

THE NATIONAL ACADEMIES PRESS
Washington, D.C.
www.nap.edu

THE NATIONAL ACADEMIES PRESS   500 Fifth Street, NW   Washington, DC 20001

NOTICE: The workshop that is the subject of this workshop summary was approved by the Governing Board of the National Research Council, whose members are drawn from the councils of the National Academy of Sciences, the National Academy of Engineering, and the Institute of Medicine.

This activity was supported by contracts between the National Academy of Sciences and the Bill & Melinda Gates Foundation, the Doris Duke Charitable Foundation, the Wellcome Trust, and the William and Flora Hewlett Foundation. The views presented in this publication do not necessarily reflect the views of the organizations or agencies that provided support for the activity.

International Standard Book Number-13: 978-0-309-30258-6
International Standard Book Number-10: 0-309-30258-7

Additional copies of this workshop summary are available for sale from the National Academies Press, 500 Fifth Street, NW, Keck 360, Washington, DC 20001; (800) 624-6242 or (202) 334-3313; http://www.nap.edu.

For more information about the Institute of Medicine, visit the IOM home page at: **www.iom.edu**.

Suggested citation: IOM (Institute of Medicine). 2014. *Evaluation design for complex global initiatives: Workshop summary.* Washington, DC: The National Academies Press.

"Knowing is not enough; we must apply.
Willing is not enough; we must do."
—Goethe

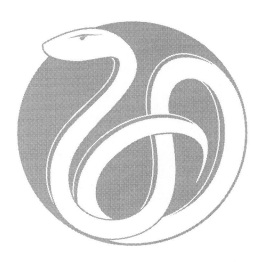

INSTITUTE OF MEDICINE
OF THE NATIONAL ACADEMIES

Advising the Nation. Improving Health.

THE NATIONAL ACADEMIES
Advisers to the Nation on Science, Engineering, and Medicine

The **National Academy of Sciences** is a private, nonprofit, self-perpetuating society of distinguished scholars engaged in scientific and engineering research, dedicated to the furtherance of science and technology and to their use for the general welfare. Upon the authority of the charter granted to it by the Congress in 1863, the Academy has a mandate that requires it to advise the federal government on scientific and technical matters. Dr. Ralph J. Cicerone is president of the National Academy of Sciences.

The **National Academy of Engineering** was established in 1964, under the charter of the National Academy of Sciences, as a parallel organization of outstanding engineers. It is autonomous in its administration and in the selection of its members, sharing with the National Academy of Sciences the responsibility for advising the federal government. The National Academy of Engineering also sponsors engineering programs aimed at meeting national needs, encourages education and research, and recognizes the superior achievements of engineers. Dr. C. D. Mote, Jr., is president of the National Academy of Engineering.

The **Institute of Medicine** was established in 1970 by the National Academy of Sciences to secure the services of eminent members of appropriate professions in the examination of policy matters pertaining to the health of the public. The Institute acts under the responsibility given to the National Academy of Sciences by its congressional charter to be an adviser to the federal government and, upon its own initiative, to identify issues of medical care, research, and education. Dr. Harvey V. Fineberg is president of the Institute of Medicine.

The **National Research Council** was organized by the National Academy of Sciences in 1916 to associate the broad community of science and technology with the Academy's purposes of furthering knowledge and advising the federal government. Functioning in accordance with general policies determined by the Academy, the Council has become the principal operating agency of both the National Academy of Sciences and the National Academy of Engineering in providing services to the government, the public, and the scientific and engineering communities. The Council is administered jointly by both Academies and the Institute of Medicine. Dr. Ralph J. Cicerone and Dr. C. D. Mote, Jr., are chair and vice chair, respectively, of the National Research Council.

www.national-academies.org

PLANNING COMMITTEE FOR THE WORKSHOP ON EVALUATING LARGE-SCALE, COMPLEX, MULTI-NATIONAL GLOBAL HEALTH INITIATIVES[1]

ANN KURTH (*Chair*), New York University, New York, NY
GEORGE ALLEYNE, Pan American Health Organization, Washington, DC
KARA HANSON, London School of Hygiene & Tropical Medicine, London, United Kingdom
DOROTHY MUROKI, FHI 360, Nairobi, Kenya
JONATHON SIMON, Boston University, Boston, MA
MARTIN VAESSEN, ICF International, Rockville, MD

IOM Staff

BRIDGET B. KELLY, Project Co-Director
KIMBERLY A. SCOTT, Project Co-Director
KATE MECK, Associate Program Officer
CHARLEE ALEXANDER, Senior Program Assistant (*from November 2013*)
JULIE WILTSHIRE, Financial Officer
PATRICK W. KELLEY, Senior Board Director, Board on Global Health

---

[1] Institute of Medicine planning committees are solely responsible for organizing the workshop, identifying topics, and choosing speakers. The responsibility for the published workshop summary rests with the workshop rapporteur and the institution.

Reviewers

This workshop summary has been reviewed in draft form by individuals chosen for their diverse perspectives and technical expertise, in accordance with procedures approved by the National Research Council's Report Review Committee. The purpose of this independent review is to provide candid and critical comments that will assist the institution in making its published workshop summary as sound as possible and to ensure that the workshop summary meets institutional standards for objectivity, evidence, and responsiveness to the study charge. The review comments and draft manuscript remain confidential to protect the integrity of the process. We wish to thank the following individuals for their review of this workshop summary:

RICHARD BERK, University of Pennsylvania
ANN KURTH, New York University
DOROTHY MUROKI, FHI 360,
SANJEEV SRIDHARAN, University of Toronto
HOWARD WHITE, International Initiative for Impact Evaluation (3ie)

Although the reviewers listed above have provided many constructive comments and suggestions, they did not see the final draft of the workshop summary before its release. The review of this workshop summary was overseen by **Enriqueta Bond**, President Emeritus, Burroughs Wellcome Fund. Appointed by the Institute of Medicine, she was responsible for making certain that an independent examination of this workshop summary was carried out in accordance with institutional procedures and that all review comments were carefully considered. Responsibility for the final content of this workshop summary rests entirely with the rapporteur and the institution.

Acknowledgments

The planning committee and project staff deeply appreciate many valuable contributions from individuals who assisted us with this project. First, we offer our profound thanks to all of the presenters and discussants at the workshop, who gave so generously of their time and expertise. These individuals are listed in full in the workshop agenda in Appendix B. We are also grateful to the many participants who attended the workshop both in person and via the live webcast. The engagement of all those in attendance was robust and vital to the success of the event. We are also particularly appreciative of the thoughtful and creative contributions of Mary Ellen Kelly and James Kelly, who applied their many years of experience to help generate the fictional initiative used for the hypothetical design exercise at the workshop.

In addition, we thank the sponsors of this project for their support: the Bill & Melinda Gates Foundation, the Doris Duke Charitable Foundation, the Wellcome Trust, and the William and Flora Hewlett Foundation. We are also grateful to the Wellcome Trust for hosting the workshop, with a special thanks to Zoe Storey, Danielle Taplin, and all of the staff there for their gracious assistance in support of every aspect of the event. We also extend many thanks to Anthony Mavrogiannis and the staff at Kentlands Travel for supporting the travel needs and requirements of this project. We appreciate LeAnn Locher's creative work in designing the report cover. Finally, we convey our gratitude for the hard work of the many staff of the Institute of Medicine and the National Academies who supported the project at every stage, from its inception to the workshop to the final production of this workshop summary report.

Contents

1

Introduction and Overview
of the Workshop[1]

Every year, public and private funders spend many billions of dollars on large-scale, complex, multi-national health initiatives. The only way to know whether these initiatives are achieving their objectives is through evaluations that examine the links between program activities and desired outcomes. Investments in such evaluations, which, like the initiatives being evaluated, are carried out in some of the world's most challenging settings, are a relatively new phenomenon. As such, it is worthwhile to reflect on the evaluations themselves to examine whether they are reaching credible, useful conclusions and how their performance can be improved.

In the last 5 years, evaluations have been conducted to determine the effects of some of the world's largest and most complex multi-national health initiatives. On January 7–8, 2014, the Institute of Medicine (IOM) held a workshop at the Wellcome Trust in London to explore these recent evaluation experiences and to consider the lessons learned from how these evaluations were designed, carried out, and used. The statement of task for the workshop can be found in Appendix A. The workshop brought together more than 100 evaluators, researchers in the field of evaluation

---

[1] The planning committee's role was limited to planning the workshop. The workshop summary has been prepared by the workshop rapporteur (with the assistance of Charlee Alexander, Bridget Kelly, Kate Meck, and Kimberly Scott) as a factual summary of what occurred at the workshop. Statements, recommendations, and opinions expressed are those of individual presenters and participants; they are not necessarily endorsed or verified by the Institute of Medicine, and they should not be construed as reflecting any group consensus.

science, staff involved in implementing large-scale health programs, local stakeholders in the countries where the initiatives are carried out, policy makers involved in the initiatives, representatives of donor organizations, and others to derive lessons learned from past large-scale evaluations and to discuss how to apply these lessons to future evaluations. The workshop was sponsored by the Bill & Melinda Gates Foundation, the Doris Duke Charitable Foundation, the Wellcome Trust, and the William and Flora Hewlett Foundation.

This workshop did not attempt to provide a comprehensive review of the rich body of literature on program evaluation theory or practice (Berk and Rossi, 1999; Leeuw and Vaessen, 2009; Rogers, 2008; Rossi et al., 2004; Royse et al., 2009; Stern et al., 2012; White and Phillips, 2012), but the evaluation examples that were examined drew on an expansive array of the available evaluation methodologies and applied them in different ways to the large-scale, complex, multi-national health initiatives. As a result, they have produced a large body of experience and knowledge that can benefit evaluations of health and development initiatives. The workshop looked at transferable insights gained across the spectrum of choosing the evaluator, framing the evaluation, designing the evaluation, gathering and analyzing data, synthesizing findings and recommendations, and communicating key messages. The workshop explored the relative benefits and limitations of different quantitative and qualitative approaches within the mixed methods designs used for these complex and costly evaluations. It was an unprecedented opportunity to capture, examine, and disseminate expert knowledge in applying evaluation science to large-scale, complex programs.

This workshop report summarizes the presentations and discussions at the workshop and is intended to convey what transpired to those involved or affected by large-scale, multi-national health initiatives, including implementers, stakeholders, evaluators, and funders of initiatives and evaluations.

TERMS AND OBJECTIVES

In her opening remarks at the workshop, Ann Kurth, professor of nursing, medicine, and public health at New York University and chair of the planning committee for the workshop, offered how the terms used in the workshop's name were being applied:

- *Large-scale*—The total cumulative budgets over multiple years amounting to at least hundreds of millions of U.S. dollars
- *Multi-national*—Implementation on a global scale, including multiple countries and regions or subregions of the world

- *Complex*
  - o Encompassing multiple components, such as varied types of interventions and programs implemented in varied settings, systems-strengthening efforts, capacity building, and efforts to influence policy change
  - o Implementation at varied levels within partner countries through a large number of diverse, multisectoral partners, including an emphasis on local governments and nongovernmental institutions

Evaluations of four large-scale, complex, multi-national health initiatives acted as core examples for the workshop:

- Global Fund to Fight AIDS, Tuberculosis, and Malaria (GF) (Sherry et al., 2009)
- U.S. President's Malaria Initiative (PMI) (Simon et al., 2011)
- Affordable Medicines Facility–malaria (AMFm) (Tougher et al., 2012)
- U.S President's Emergency Plan for AIDS Relief (PEPFAR) (IOM, 2013)

Appendix C provides a comparison of the evaluations for these initiatives. In addition, the workshop examined other evaluations of large-scale health and development initiatives along with smaller-scale evaluations that share similar features of complexity.

Evaluations need to be credible, rigorous, feasible, affordable, and matched to the priority evaluation questions, aims, and audiences, Kurth said. No single evaluation design can serve every purpose, and every evaluation must make strategic choices that fit its context and goals. But the process of designing and conducting an evaluation has key strategic decision-making points, and the available choices have different advantages and disadvantages that result in trade-offs for any given design decision. Evaluations of complex initiatives require more complicated strategic design considerations, but many of the issues discussed at the workshop are applicable to evaluations all along the spectrum of complexity.

Though the workshop sought to identify lessons learned, it was not designed to look backward, said Kurth. Rather, the underlying objective was to be "candid, open, and frank" about past experiences to create a foundation for future improvements.

MESSAGES FROM THE WORKSHOP

In the final session of the workshop, some of the important messages over the previous 2 days were recapitulated by three experienced evaluators (Chapter 12 provides a full account of their remarks):

1. Sanjeev Sridharan, director of the Evaluation Centre for Complex Health Interventions at Li Ka Shing Knowledge Institute at St. Michaels Hospital and associate professor in the Department of Health Policy, Management, and Evaluation at the University of Toronto;
2. Charlotte Watts, head of the Social and Mathematical Epidemiology Group and founding director of the Gender, Violence, and Health Centre in the Department for Global Health and Development at the London School of Hygiene and Tropical Medicine; and
3. Elliot Stern, emeritus professor of evaluation research at Lancaster University and visiting professor at Bristol University.

The workshop then closed with reflections from representatives of the four funders of the workshop— Gina Dallabetta of the Bill & Melinda Gates Foundation, Mary Bassett of the Doris Duke Charitable Foundation, Jimmy Whitworth of the Wellcome Trust, and Ruth Levine of the William and Flora Hewlett Foundation—on the major lessons and messages they were taking away from the event.

The following messages of the workshop are drawn from these speaker's remarks. These should not be seen as recommendations or conclusions emerging from the workshop, but they provide a useful summary of some of the major topics discussed.

What Evaluations Can Do

Evaluations typically have multiple objectives, said Charlotte Watts, head of the Social and Mathematical Epidemiology Group and founding director of the Gender, Violence, and Health Centre in the Department for Global Health and Development at the London School of Hygiene and Tropical Medicine. Some evaluations are focused specifically on assessing an intervention's impact and cost-effectiveness, but others have broader public good aspects. An evaluation may also aim to derive lessons about scaling up or replicating effective interventions, build capacity for evaluations, or strengthen networks of researchers and practitioners.

Ruth Levine, director of the Global Development and Population Program at the William and Flora Hewlett Foundation Evaluations, commented that evaluations are used to hold governments, funders, and other stakeholders accountable for the use of the resources that are dedicated to large initiatives that have proliferated and have high political visibility. Similarly, Jimmy Whitworth, head of population health at the Wellcome Trust, notes that policy makers have been challenging the public health community to learn more about the effects of its interventions as a way to justify and increase investments in large-scale initiatives. To that end, evaluations of public health investments may inform not only program improvements, but also policy and funding decisions.

Sanjeev Sridharan, director of the Evaluation Centre for Complex Health Interventions at Li Ka Shing Knowledge Institute at St. Michaels Hospital and associate professor in the Department of Health Policy, Management, and Evaluation at the University of Toronto observed that very few large-scale, complex, multi-national initiatives are well formed from their earliest stages and noted that evaluations can also contribute to the development of an initiative. This may require a changing relationship with evaluators over time, but it can build capacity in both the evaluation and the initiative that can lead to continual improvements.

Governance and Evaluator Independence

Gina Dallabetta, a program officer at the Bill & Melinda Gates Foundation, appreciated that the workshop focused on the larger view of evaluation, including issues such as governance. In particular, the question of how independent evaluators should be was raised by several of the participants. These initiatives are incentivized to claim success so that they can maintain high levels of resources and political commitment, Levine noted. On the other hand, Sridharan noted that program staff are generally among the most critical observers of their programs. It does not take a faraway researcher to be objective. Sridharan proposed a nuanced position with degrees of independence depending on the phase and intent of the evaluation. For an evaluation early in a project, a close relationship with an evaluator may allow for valuable input to program staff as they design or modify an intervention. A results-focused evaluation may need to achieve more independence from a program to deliver unbiased results. Elliot Stern, emeritus professor of evaluation research at Lancaster University and visiting professor at Bristol University, added that it may be possible to have different people involved in different evaluation phases to obtain the appropriate levels of independence.

Evaluation Framing and Design

Evaluations need to prioritize the questions they are asking, said Levine, which means thinking through the kinds of questions that could change the minds of decision makers, whether within the program or at a higher level. Watts stated that understanding program effectiveness cannot be reduced to answering a closed-ended question about whether "it worked." Perhaps the evaluation questions should be more nuanced: Can you do it at scale? Can you do it with this population? Can you sustain it? This provides a greater space for the framing of questions, the evaluation design, and for partnership between evaluators and program staff.

A wealth of techniques and methodologies are available for evaluation, but the strength of an evaluation lies in careful design. Many of the speakers highlighted that an underlying initial step is to articulate an underlying program theory or similar framework to understand the fundamental assumptions that need to be interrogated. Watts emphasized the importance of designing a mixed methods approach to achieve a full understanding of a large-scale, complex, multi-national initiative. Qualitative and quantitative work can be nested in parallel, and qualitative and quantitative data can be triangulated to increase confidence in the evidence base for evaluation findings.

Understanding Context

The evaluators emphasized the critical importance for evaluation design of understanding the relationship between context and the desired outcomes for intervention and evaluation designs. Sridharan noted it is best to bring the knowledge of context in at the start, but also to understand how it is evolving and adapting over time. Mary Bassett of the Doris Duke Charitable Foundation Evaluators reiterated the need to devote heightened attention to context, referring to how Elliot Stern in his comments "really challenged us to unpack the notion of what context means." Contextual issues arise on micro-, meso-, and macro-scales, and all can be important. Droughts, economic crises, and political changes are some factors that can affect the outcome of an initiative and should be tracked, but it is also important to think about how to understand issues of leadership, power, trust, communication, and community engagement that have all been talked about, Bassett said.

Data Availability and Quality

Many types of data collection can be prospectively embedded within a program for evaluation. Gina Dallabetta, a program officer at the Bill & Melinda Gates Foundation, emphasized strengthening capacity for quality data collection in countries, especially as projects become larger and more complex. Dallabetta noted that program evaluations can be hampered by a lack of quality routine data collected within countries, reflecting a need for management expertise to help countries collect better data, including process data, outcome data, and financial data. These data can be used for both program monitoring by management and evaluation, but data collection and analysis need to be based on a theory of change before program implementation begins, said Dallabetta.

However, evaluators also need to do original data collection to have ways to validate the data reported by programs, Levine said. She also observed that many more sources of nontraditional data will be available in the future, such as geospatial analyses, citizen feedback, transactional data about what people are purchasing and where they are going, and sensors such as smart pill bottles.

All four of the workshop funders emphasized the importance of open data, so that the information on which conclusions are based is available to others. Levine noted that if data can be made available to others for reanalysis, this can reinforce technical quality. Dallabetta added, however, that data sometimes belong to governments or have multiple owners, which may require that one centralized place exist in a country where people can view data. Maintaining open data also requires work, such as data archiving and documentation, that donors need to build into their funding.

Using the Results of Evaluations

Though the use of an evaluation's results can be one of the factors least in control of an evaluation team, evaluators can enhance the use of their results in a variety of ways, said Levine. An especially promising approach is to meaningfully engage a wide range of stakeholders in an ongoing way. Evaluators also can encourage systematic follow-up of recommendations, in part by creating a culture of learning versus one of punishment. Evaluations need adequate planning, skills, and budgets for a fit-for-purpose dissemination, Levine said. Whitworth observed that the public health community also needs to do a better job of celebrating and publicizing its successes as a way of increasing support for large-scale programs. Large-scale, complex, multi-national initiatives have produced some of the biggest success stories of international health and development assistance, and those stories have been backed up by credible evidence, said Levine. Watts similarly observed that strong evaluations require resources, commitment, investments, trust, and strong relationships, but they can be tremendously beneficial for public health.

Final Reflections on Future Large-Scale, Complex Evaluations

As part of the workshop's final session, Levine shared some thoughts about future evaluations of large-scale, complex, multi-national initiatives as well as other evaluations that will benefit from the information shared at the workshop.

One important lesson derived from recent large-scale initiatives is how to increase the space for serious evaluations, said Levine. The public health community has a tradition of basing program design on good evidence and then learning as it goes based on additional evidence. "The potential for evaluations to actually make a difference is there," said Levine, also observing that improving the technical quality of evaluations is a demanding task.

One important trend that will influence future evaluations is a new partnership model with the countries in which programs are being implemented and evaluated. Evaluations need mandates from governments and donors doing rigorous work, Levine observed, and they need the funding to be able to do that work. At the same time, evaluations need the governance and advisory structures to be insulated from political influence.

The advocacy community can support evaluations in this regard by praising initiatives that not only do evaluations but then make use of findings to correct shortcomings. "The very same advocates who are so good at pushing for more money for global health programs can, and sometimes have been, very capable advocates for evaluating and using the findings from evaluations for more effective programming," said Levine.

Another trend that will make itself felt in the future is an increase in "uninvited co-evaluators." Many people have access to evaluation information who have an interest in challenging not just the program but the evaluation. As Levine said, "There is a lower barrier to entry into the conversation, and that is in some abstract way a positive thing, [but] in the day-to-day reality, it's very challenging."

Finally, Levine closed with a list of potential activities or steps for improvement for evaluators and funders:

Evaluators

- Document the stories of evaluations.
- Create greater value in global collaborations.
- Be honest about the feasibility of sponsors' demands.
- Participate in method development and validation.
- Connect with the evaluation community outside of the health sector.
- Train the next generation.
- Embrace transparency.

Funders

- Create incentives for learning.
- Make reasonable demands of evaluators, and fund at the right level.
- Permit or require transparency.

ORGANIZATION OF THE WORKSHOP REPORT

Following this introductory chapter, Chapter 2 of this summary of the workshop describes an overview framework for evaluation design, introducing many of the topics discussed at the workshop.

Chapters 3–8 are arranged to present the major components of design and implementation in roughly the sequence that they might be addressed during the course of an evaluation, although each evaluation is different and many of these components are typically addressed or re-addressed iteratively and continuously throughout the evaluation process.

Chapter 3 discusses how evaluations are framed when choosing the evaluator, establishing the governance structure of the evaluation, and developing and prioritizing the evaluation questions. Chapter 4 examines the development of an evaluation's design and particularly the methodological choices and trade-offs evaluators must make in the design process. Chapter 5 considers data sources and the processes of gathering and assessing data.

Chapters 6 and 7, which are drawn from two of four concurrent sessions that were held during the workshop, examine methodological and data issues in more detail. Chapter 6 looks at the application of qualitative methods to evaluation on a large scale, while Chapter 7 does the same for quantitative methods. Chapter 8 then turns to the use of triangulation and synthesis in analyzing data from multiple data sources and across multiple methods to yield a deeper and richer perspective on an initiative and increase confidence in the evidence base for evaluation findings.

Chapters 9 and 10, which are drawn from the other two workshop concurrent sessions, explore specific extensions of some of the ideas discussed earlier in the workshop. Chapter 9 looks at evolving methods in evaluation science, including realist methods and nonexperimental, observational, and mixed methods. Chapter 10 discusses how principles that are important for large-scale program evaluations can similarly be applied to complex evaluations on a smaller scale. Chapter 11 then examines how the findings and key messages of an evaluation are used and can be disseminated to diverse audiences. In Chapter 12, three experienced evaluators reflect on the messages of the workshop and how they might apply to future evaluations through the lens of a hypothetical evaluation design exercise for a fictional multi-national initiative.

2

Overview Framework for Complex Evaluations

Important Points Made by the Speaker

- Interventions can vary in complexity along different dimensions.
- Many methods are available to describe the implementation of an intervention, to acquire data about an intervention's effects, and to assess the contribution to or attribution of impact.
- Many methods are complex and rapidly changing, creating a demand for guidance in their use.

In the opening session of the workshop, Simon Hearn, a research fellow at the Overseas Development Institute, set the stage for discussing the practice of designing and implementing mixed methods evaluations of large complex interventions and presented an overall framework for approaching these types of evaluations. He described the BetterEvaluation Initiative, a global collaboration of many organizations dedicated to improving evaluation practice and theory.[1]

Hearn identified three major challenges in evaluating complex interventions:

1. Describing what is being implemented
2. Getting data about impacts
3. Attributing impacts to a particular program

---

[1] More information is available at http://betterevaluation.org (accessed April 7, 2014).

Many different evaluation methods are available to take on these challenges, as are guides for how to do evaluations. But many methods are evolving rapidly, and new methods and data sources are becoming available, such as the use of mobile phones or social media. Also, options exist for understanding causality that do not involve experimental methods, though these are often not covered in guides. In such circumstances, evaluators often use the methods they have always used, said Hearn, which may or may not be suited to the problem at hand.

Hearn also discussed six facets of interventions that, when viewed together, can be used to gauge the complexity of an intervention:

1. Objectives: Are they clear and defined ahead of time, or are they emergent and changing over time?
2. Governance: Is it clear and defined ahead of time, or is it characterized by shifting responsibilities and networks of actors?
3. Implementation: Is the implementation of the intervention consistent across places and across time, or will it shift and change over time?
4. Necessariness: Is the intervention the only thing necessary for its intended impacts, or do other pathways lead to the impacts, and are these pathways knowable?
5. Sufficiency: Is the intervention sufficient to achieve the impacts, or do other factors need to be in place for the impacts to be realized, and are these other factors predictable before the fact?
6. Change trajectory: Is the change trajectory straightforward? Can the relationship between inputs and outcomes be defined, and will this relationship change over time?

THE BETTEREVALUATION INITIATIVE RAINBOW FRAMEWORK

Hearn and his colleagues have developed the BetterEvaluation Rainbow Framework to help evaluators navigate the choices available at each stage of an evaluation (see Figure 2-1). The framework organizes clusters of tasks associated with each stage of the evaluation process, although the stages and tasks are not necessarily sequential, and each is as valuable as the other. Furthermore, all are subject to management, which acts as a sort of prism through which all the different stages of an overall evaluation process are viewed.

The *first task* is to define what is to be evaluated. This involves developing an initial description of the initiative or program being evaluated (the evaluand), developing a program theory or logic model to describe how the program is intended to create change, and identifying potential unintended results. For example, a logic model may consist of a simple pipeline

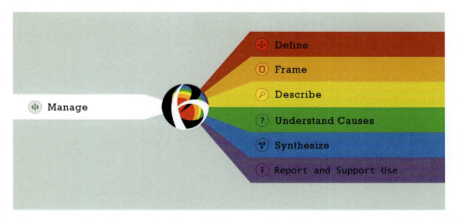

FIGURE 2-1 BetterEvaluation Initiative's Rainbow Framework, as presented by Hearn, separates an evaluation into equally important tasks that each need to be managed.
SOURCE: BetterEvaluation, 2014.

or results chain, a more sophisticated logical framework, more structured and free-flowing outcomes hierarchies, or realist matrices, though complex evaluations are much more likely to rely on the more sophisticated models. Prominent questions include whether an evaluation is looking at the effects on policy, the effects on populations, or both; whether multiple levels of activity are being evaluated; and who the stakeholders are. A clear description can engage and inform all of the stakeholders involved in the evaluation, Hearn said, which is particularly important in complex evaluations where many people are involved.

The *second task* is to frame what is to be evaluated. Framing an evaluation is necessary to design that evaluation. Framing involves identifying the primary intended users, deciding on the purposes of the evaluation, specifying key evaluation questions, and determining what "success" would look like—what standards or criteria will be used to make judgments about the program? Complex interventions are likely to have multiple contributors and users of results, and Hearn noted that the different purposes of these users can conflict. Users also may have different evaluation questions that need to be addressed, which means they might have different understandings of success.

The *third task* is to describe what happened. This task involves the use of samples, measures, or indicators; the collection and management of data; the combination of qualitative and quantitative data; the analysis of data; and the visualization and communication of data. For example, in combining qualitative and quantitative data, the purposes of the combination need to be examined, whether enriching the quantitative data with qualitative data or examining hypotheses emerging from qualitative analysis with quantitative analysis. Similarly, do unexpected quantitative results need to be explained with qualitative information, or do particular results need to be "triangulated" to verify or reject a conclusion? (The issue of triangulation is discussed in Chapter 6.) Are data from one phase of a project being used to inform another phase? Are the data being gathered in parallel or in sequence? Many different options are available in this area, said Hearn.

The *fourth task* is to understand the causes of outcomes and impacts. What caused particular impacts, and did an intervention contribute to those outcomes? Do the results support causal attributions? How do the results compare with the counterfactual analysis? What alternative explanations are possible? Simply collecting information about what happened cannot answer questions about causes and effects, whereas an evaluation must deal with causation in some way, Hearn observed. Evaluations often either oversimplify or overcomplicate this process. Oversimplification can come from an implicit assumption that if something is observed it can be understood as caused by the program or interventions—making a "leap of faith" without doing the analysis to verify the claim. Overcomplication can lead to overly elaborate experimental designs or to the analysis of very large datasets with overly sophisticated statistical techniques. Experimental designs can be powerful, but other options are also available, and causation can be measured even without control groups or experimentation. Theory-based designs, participatory designs, counterfactual analysis, regulatory frameworks, configurational frameworks, generative frameworks, realist evaluation, general elimination method, process tracing, contribution analysis, and qualitative comparative analysis are among the many techniques that can explore causation. Indeed, said Hearn, the BetterEvaluation website has 29 different options for understanding causes.

The *fifth task* is to synthesize data to make overall judgments about the worth of an intervention. Among the many questions that can be asked at this stage are: Was it good? Did it work? Was it effective? For whom did it work? In what ways did it work? Did it provide value for money? Was it cost-effective? Synthesis can occur at the micro level, the meso level, and the macro level. At the micro level, performance on particular dimensions is assessed. At the meso level, different individual assessments can be synthesized to answer evaluation questions. At the macro level, the merit or worth of an intervention can be assessed.

Synthesis can look at a single evaluation or at multiple evaluations, and it can generalize findings from, for example, a small population to a larger population. Synthesis can be difficult in cases where some positive and some negative impacts have been achieved, which requires weighing up the strengths and weaknesses of the interventions. But synthesis is essential for evaluations, said Hearn, even though it is often slighted or overlooked in textbooks and research designs.

The *sixth task* is to report results and support use. "We are in the business of evaluation because we want those evaluations to make a difference," said Hearn. "We do not want them just to be published as a report and for the users of those reports to ignore them or to misuse them." This task requires identifying reporting requirements for different stakeholders; developing reporting media, whether written reports, social media campaigns, or some other output; ensuring accessibility for those who can use the results; developing recommendations where appropriate; and helping users of evaluations to apply the findings.

Finally, Hearn discussed the management of these six tasks, which includes but is not limited to the following elements:

- Understand and engage with stakeholders.
- Establish decision-making processes.
- Decide who will conduct the evaluation.
- Determine and secure resources.
- Define ethical and quality evaluation standards.
- Document management processes and agreements.
- Develop an evaluation plan or framework.
- Review the evaluation.
- Develop evaluation capacity.

These management tasks are relevant throughout the entire process of the evaluation, applying to each of the previous tasks.

NAVIGATING THE FRAMEWORK

Hearn provided three tips to help evaluators navigate the framework, which is available on the BetterEvaluation website.[2] The first tip is to look at the types of questions being asked, whether descriptive, causal, synthetic, or use oriented. For example, a descriptive question is whether the policy was implemented as planned; a causal question is whether a policy contributed to improved health outcomes; a synthetic question is whether the overall policy was a success; and a use-oriented question is what should be done. The question being asked will determine which part of the framework to access.

The second tip is to compare the pros and cons of each possible

---

[2] More information is available at http://betterevaluation.org (accessed April 7, 2014).

method. The website provides methods and resources for each of the six tasks, and this information can be used to select the optimal method.

The third tip is to create a two-dimensional evaluation matrix that has the key evaluation questions along one side and the methods along the other. By filling out this matrix, a toolkit can be developed to match questions with the methods that will be used to answer those questions.

The website offers much more information on each of the elements of the framework, as well as other resources. The BetterEvaluation organization also runs events, clinics, workshops, and other events to help teams work through evaluation design, and it then feeds the information generated by such experiences into its website. In addition, it issues publications and other forms of guidance and information.

The vision of the BetterEvaluation initiative, Hearn concluded, is to foster collaborations to produce more information and more guidance on methods to improve evaluation. The topic and the structure of this workshop are aligned to the principles of the framework, Hearn observed, and it is an opportunity to "push us further" to fill gaps and work together for a "better understanding of the richness and variety of methods" for evaluation.

3

Framing the Evaluation

Important Points Made by the Speakers

- By prioritizing and organizing the questions to be addressed by evaluations into manageable units, realistic instruments and a framework for conducting the evaluation can be designed.
- Evaluations require that trade-offs be made along a number of dimensions, including the balance of independence and interdependence.
- Multiple goals for an evaluation may not be incompatible but often require different approaches.
- Evaluations can enhance their value by building in-country capacity and by involving more local participants in the evaluation.

Any evaluation effort starts by framing the evaluation. In the workshop's opening session, five panelists discussed various approaches for this key initial step. From their individual experiences, the panelists addressed such issues as developing and prioritizing the evaluation questions, defining the audiences and intended uses for the evaluation, the relationship between the evaluators and the evaluands, and trade-offs in choosing the type of evaluator and in identifying and establishing the governance structure for an evaluation. Evaluations of large-scale, complex, multi-national initiatives are themselves going to be complex, which requires, as pointed out in the previous chapter, well-managed pursuit of discrete tasks.

REFLECTIONS FROM THE EXPERIENCE OF THE EVALUATION OF THE U.S. PRESIDENT'S MALARIA INITIATIVE

Framing an evaluation starts with a small set of well-defined questions, said workshop planning committee member and panel moderator Jonathon Simon, who is Robert A. Knox Professor and director of the Center for Global Health and Development at Boston University. What often happens, however, is that evaluators are presented with "laundry lists from smart people [who are] passionately committed to issues within agencies or organizations that want to know everything about everything." Simon gave several examples from the evaluation of the U.S. President's Malaria Initiative (PMI), noting that the initial evaluation request from the PMI included a list of 82 questions that contained another 50 or so questions nested within that list. It is essential, then, to prioritize and organize the questions in manageable units that can be used to design realistic instruments and a framework for conducting the evaluation.

It is then necessary to consider the audiences for the results of the evaluation beyond the discrete audience of those in charge of the effort being evaluated. For the evaluation of PMI, explained Simon, the *Washington Post* was an audience, as was a group of think tanks that had been criticizing the initiative. A large political audience for the evaluation was more concerned with whether the PMI was working and less interested in the technical evaluations of the interventions. Financial considerations were also a factor, given that the PMI was up for reauthorization.

Within the U.S. Agency for International Development (USAID) and the Centers for Disease Control and Prevention (CDC)—the agencies in charge of the PMI—the leaders of both organizations had substantive interest in the evaluation, but the evaluation goals of the two agencies were different. An additional consideration was that the evaluation was not mandated by Congress but was commissioned by the initiative's director. For the evaluators, an important audience was the group of people leading the country-level efforts and implementing the program on the ground. "Could we do an evaluation that actually added value or contributed to national malaria control programs, and could the country personnel actually benefit or learn from the evaluation?" Recognizing the ways in which the results will be reported and used and the legitimate needs of the different audiences for an evaluation points to the complexity of designing an evaluation, said Simon.

Regarding the relationship between the evaluators and the evaluand, Simon said that the reason he was asked to conduct the evaluation was that he was perceived to be independent of the "malaria mafia." While that was the case, Simon said that the evaluation was funded by grants from USAID, CDC, and other agencies of the U.S. government. To maintain the objectivity of the evaluation team, Simon insisted on operational independence. "We took control of the process once the original framing was done, and we had a set of agreements that the agencies would not see anything until they received a draft report," he said. While it was important to maintain operational independence from the funders of the evaluation, Simon and his colleagues often had to rely on the PMI staff to gain the cooperation of the in-country teams. To illustrate that objectivity required a balance between independence and interdependence, Simon explained that while the evaluation team received 167 comments from the funders in response to the draft report, the evaluators chose which comments to address and which to reject.

Maintaining the right balance in terms of independence and interdependence ties into the issue of trade-offs. Simon identified seven trade-offs that were made in evaluating the PMI. There were methodological trade-offs in terms of setting the right mix of qualitative and quantitative methods and the use of data from routine monitoring programs. Given that the PMI is active in 15 countries, there were geographic trade-offs; in the end, the evaluators conducted site visits in 5 countries and relied on telephone interviews in the other 10 countries, resulting in some degree of selection bias. There were trade-offs in terms of which technical interventions were assessed from a functional perspective, such as indoor residual spraying versus bed nets. Another set of trade-offs involved the priority given to the various audiences, including political, financial, programmatic, and country-level audiences. Time and money were not infinite, which also necessitated trade-offs. Finally, there is the value trade-off between the perfect design and results that are useful and informative. "How you do the value trade-off is one of the key challenges that we deal with in these large, multicountry, complex evaluations," he said in closing.

EVALUATION AT THE UNITED NATIONS

The United Nations (UN) Office of Inspection and Oversight (OID), which is one of three bodies with oversight functions at the UN, is responsible for evaluating 32 different UN programs and entities that engage in a wide range of activities, from peacekeeping operations to humanitarian and environmental programs, explained Deborah Rugg, director of the Inspection and Evaluation Division at the UN Secretariat. Her office has 22 professional evaluators on staff, largely methodologists, and it contracts with external experts for subject-matter expertise. OID reports through the UN Secretary General to the 193 member states. The fact that these evaluations are mandated gives her office both authority and funding, which makes what Rugg characterized as a huge difference in terms of participation by and cooperation from staff with the evaluated programs.

Each year, her office conducts an average of eight assessments that examine the extent to which a program has been funded, its size, how many evaluations of the program have been conducted, if there is a need for evaluation, and if there are any current topical issues germane to the need for evaluation. For example, many of the peacekeeping evaluations are based on current political and contextual issues that need urgent attention as well as the capacity within that entity to do an evaluation. She noted that at one time OID evaluations were largely for accountability purposes and offered little information in terms of value, which meant that evaluations were largely noncollaborative activities. Today, Rugg and her colleagues use a partnership model that solicits input on what needs to be evaluated to answer important operational and functional questions. This partnership approach has led to increased use of the evaluation reports, she said.

The issue of independence is an important one at the UN and for the UN evaluation group, and Rugg pointed to three levels of independence. Institutional independence means that her group operates as an independent group outside of a program without an institutional direct line of report. Operational independence means that while the evaluation of UN programs is conducted by a UN office, her group sits outside of the programs that it evaluates. Behavioral independence refers to an absence of coercion by the program being evaluated or of a conflict of interest for those conducting the evaluation. "I have to prove in all of OID's evaluations that we are not unduly influenced by the program, or more importantly, by any specific country," explained Rugg. Some programs are evaluated more frequently than others, but on average, programs can expect to be evaluated about once every 8 years, which she said is a reasonable time frame if there also are internal embedded evaluations to answer more timely and program-relevant questions. "That's one of the trade-offs with these large-scale, infrequent evaluations is that they can address high-level issues with a global context, but they cannot drill down as effectively as one might expect," she said. "We would like to see more internal evaluation capacity building so that that can answer specific questions in a more timely basis."

To increase utilization of findings, evaluations now start with a 3-month inception phase in which her office holds conversations with potential users, reviews prior evaluations, and attempts to develop a better understanding of how an evaluation can be useful to program staff as well as to the UN as a whole. After completing an evaluation, her group works with the evaluated program and conducts follow-up sessions to check on implementation of any recommendations suggested by the evaluation or that are mandated by the member states. A typical evaluation takes about 1 year, which includes the 3-month inception period followed by 3 months of data collection, 3 months of analysis and writing, and a 3-month clearance process. Rugg characterized this as a short period of time that balances a trade-off between producing actionable and timely results of a program against depth of experimental and analytic design.

In terms of the the Joint United Nations Program on HIV/AIDS (UNAIDS) program, Rugg said that ongoing internal evaluations are focusing on performance monitoring, while an external, independent evaluation is conducted every 5 years and a variety of ad hoc special evaluation studies focus on specific programmatic issues. In addition, in-country residents in regional offices around the world work to support the national governments' evaluations and capacity building.

AN EVALUATION FUNDER'S PERSPECTIVE
ON WHERE PROBLEMS ARISE

After agreeing with the points that the previous speakers had made, Christopher Whitty, chief scientific advisor at the United Kingdom's Department for International Development (DFID), noted that, in his view, program officials who work outside of the health care arena have not historically had much appreciation for the fact that "good ideas, passionately delivered by people to the highest quality, may not work." As a result, outside of health care, not much value has been placed on evaluation, though he acknowledged that this situation is changing for the better. Other positive developments, he said, include the improvement in the methodologies available for performing complex evaluations and greater acceptance that mixed methods approaches, or using both quantitative and qualitative methods for data collection and analysis, are important for evaluations.

In his role as a commissioner at DFID, Whitty is on the receiving end of evaluations and has seen a number of outstanding evaluations over the past few years, including the independent evaluation of the Affordable Medicines Facility–malaria (AMFm). Most evaluations, however, have not been outstanding, and he observed that some of the reasons are on the side of those who request and fund evaluations. The biggest problem from the donor perspective, he said, is that those who commission evaluations have multiple goals for the evaluation that, while not necessarily incompatible, actually require distinctly different approaches. One goal is to provide assurance to those who pay for a given program—the British public in his case—that their money is not being wasted. A second goal is to check on the efficacy of a program and make course corrections if needed. The third goal is impact evaluation—what about a program has worked and what has not, what has been cost-effective and what has not, and what aspects can be improved in the next iteration of the program?

The problem, said Whitty, is that those who ask for evaluations often are asking for a single evaluation that meets all three goals at the same time. "If someone asks you for all three, you have to tell them that they are different things and they are going to have to pay more and probably have to do it by at least two different mechanisms." This discussion has to take place up-front between the person who would do the evaluation and the person commissioning an evaluation to avoid wasting time and money on pointless activities, he added. Another confounding factor is that most of the large, complex programs are conceived by what Whitty characterized as "very smart, very politically connected, and very charismatic true believers." The resulting political realities have to be considered in the initial design discussions between funders and evaluators.

On the side of the evaluators, poorly performed evaluations are often the result of the difficulty of evaluating complex programs. "What we are talking about here is intrinsically difficult. Many of these things are really hard to evaluate.... I do not believe there is such a thing as perfect design for most of the things we are talking about in this meeting." He described assessing whether a design is poorly conceived based on whether he would change his mind about a program if the evaluation did not provide the answer he expected or desired. If the evaluation is not "sufficiently strong methodologically that you are forced to change your mind," he stated, then "you probably should not do the evaluation in the first place. That seems to me to be a common sense test." Another problem that he sees on the delivery side is that evaluations of complex programs require teams comprising individuals with a wide range of skills, and assembling such multidisciplinary teams is difficult. How to facilitate the formation of multidisciplinary teams is "something that we as donors as well as providers need to think through," he said.

LESSONS LEARNED FROM THE GLOBAL FUND TO FIGHT AIDS, TUBERCULOSIS, AND MALARIA

The Global Fund to Fight AIDS, Tuberculosis, and Malaria was established in 2002 as an international financing mechanism that would help countries scale up programs that were shown to be effective in pilot studies. The Technical Evaluation Reference Group (TERG) is an independent evaluation advisory group accountable to the Global Fund's board for conducting an independent evaluation of the Global Fund's business model and impact, and in November 2006 the board commissioned an evaluation after the first 5-year grant cycle. Working together, TERG and the board defined three study areas that were mutually interdependent and several overarching questions for each study area.

Ryuichi Komatsu, senior advisor for TERG at the Global Fund Secretariat, explained that the first study area focused on organizational efficiency and effectiveness and addressed the overarching question of whether the Global Fund's activities reflected its core principles, including country ownership and its actions as a financial instrument. The second study area examined whether the Global Fund's partner environment was effective and efficient. This study area addressed two overarching questions: How effective and efficient is the Global Fund partnership at the country group level? and What is the wider effect of Global Fund partnership on a country's health care delivery systems? The third study area looked at the impact of the Global Fund's programs on disease by asking if there had been an overall reduction in the incidence of AIDS, tuberculosis, and malaria and what the Global Fund's programs contributed to this reduction. TERG conducted three separate studies involving multiple countries at a cost of $16 million. The resulting evaluation, conducted by a consortia of organizations, took 3 years to complete from initial design to release of a synthesis report.

One lesson learned from this evaluation was that 3 years was a very short time frame for such a complex evaluation. As a result, Komatsu explained, there was little time for aligning the evaluation with in-country processes such as annual health department reviews or conducting national surveys. In addition, the short time frame resulted in some in-country task forces not being fully engaged in the evaluation process. Nonetheless, the Global Fund has used the results of the evaluation to create a new funding model that has been launched recently, and it has taken steps to address the evaluation's shortcomings by emphasizing continuous smaller country-level evaluations on which to build comprehensive evaluations that can better inform ongoing grant management at the country level. This new model also reduces the logistical challenge of evaluating multiple countries, each with its own operational cycle, simultaneously.

To evaluate the impact of program scale in specific countries, TERG has decided to rely on country health-sector reviews and disease program reviews in the context of national strategies. These reviews are assisted by the World Health Organization (WHO) and UNAIDS, and they are conducted by a team of independent experts. "Results from such reviews can be practical and immediately fit into the management of grants, especially in the context of the new funding model of the Global Fund," explained Komatsu. While it is challenging to achieve and maintain consistent quality across countries, TERG has been working with WHO to strengthen the guidance for these reviews, and it also has commissioned an independent consultant to conduct a midterm review of this evaluation strategy.

Finally, Komatsu explained that TERG now emphasizes five key principles in designing its evaluations: periodic, plausibility design, country platform, practicality, and partner approach, which means to build on, collaborate, and align evaluations with partners while maintaining and ensuring rigor and objectivity.

COMPARING EVALUATIONS OF SELECTED GLOBAL INITIATIVES

Robert Black, professor and director of the Institute for International Programs in the Department of International Health at the Johns Hopkins Bloomberg School of Public Health, compared the goals and approaches used to evaluate five different global initiatives with which he has been involved. He started by comparing the Global Fund evaluation discussed by Komatsu with the evaluation of the U.S. President's Emergency Plan for AIDS Relief (PEPFAR). While the Global Fund evaluation looked at selected countries in the program and presented results for each country, the PEPFAR evaluation looked at the program as a whole and did not report country-specific findings. Another difference between the two evaluations was time frame—the PEPFAR evaluation was conducted over 4 years, which led to challenges in dealing with a program that was evolving as the evaluation was being conducted. Both evaluations focused on program performance, though the PEPFAR evaluation had a particular focus on prevention, care, and treatment targets as well as on how the initiative affected local health systems. In terms of who conducted the evaluation, the Global Fund's effort was overseen by TERG and conducted by a consortium of five institutions working with in-country institutions. The PEPFAR study was conducted by the Institute of Medicine (IOM) as mandated by the U.S. Congress. Two IOM committees with the majority of members overlapping were involved in the study: one for planning, the other for implementation (IOM, 2013; IOM and NRC, 2010).

In Black's opinion, the Global Fund's evaluations made trade-offs among country ownership, objectivity, and independence of the assessment and among rigor, timeliness, and capacity building. For PEPFAR, Black emphasized what was in his view an unfortunate trade-off: not being able to report findings that were specific to individual countries, which was due to the framing of the original evaluation mandate and to the necessity of assuring country de-identification to receive secondary quantitative data and to maximize candor in qualitative data collection. As far as independence and objectivity in the PEPFAR study, Black said that the IOM is very strong on avoiding conflict of interest among committee members, and the process was developed and carried out with complete independence, with the sponsoring organization not receiving the report until it was finalized after extensive review by outside experts. In terms of the data collection, the qualitative data were independently collected, but for the quantitative data the evaluation relied heavily on the data from the program implementers.

The Integrated Management of Childhood Illness (IMCI) initiative evaluation was a prospective evaluation of effort in 60 nations that was conducted by a WHO advisory committee and in-country institutions with funding from the Bill & Melinda Gates Foundation. In this case, explained

Black, the UN agency responsible for the program also was responsible for the evaluation, and its focus was on quality of care, feasibility, and costs. For the IMCI assessment, the evaluation was limited to five countries selected by WHO that were thought to have the strongest implementation in order to assess the impact of the program on health. Though the evaluation was conducted by the implementing agency, there was a strong, independent advisory committee.

The retrospective evaluation of the Accelerated Child Survival and Development Program (ACSD), which operated in 11 West African nations, focused on quality of care, feasibility, costs, and in particular the impact of the program on child mortality; it was funded by Canada through the UN Children's Fund (UNICEF). The ACSD evaluation was limited to countries that UNICEF claimed were benefiting from the program. "The fact that the independent evaluation did not find that made us very unpopular," said Black. "Therefore, there was a great degree of discomfort with the independence of the evaluation."

The ongoing evaluation of the 10-country Millennium Village initiative is looking at feasibility, cost, and achievement of program goals. However, there has been some concern, said Black, because the evaluation is being done by the program itself. There is an advisory committee, which he chairs, and their role is evolving. This evaluation is still being finalized and planned, he noted.

All of these evaluations, Black said, had the intent of measuring both program performance and health impact, which he characterized as a good thing. However, the feasibility and the timeline for these evaluations need to be questioned and thought through thoroughly, he said. He noted, too, that some aspects of country selection may compromise the generalizability and representativeness of the evaluation findings, and he reiterated his belief that there should be some obligation to provide feedback to the countries. He said that issues related to funding of the implementation of an evaluation also need to be thought through carefully. "In all of the examples I have seen, funding is linked in some strong way with the program, which to me compromises independence." Black commented that the evaluations he described almost all have some kind of trade-off in their framing and design that limits what kind of evaluation can be done, for example, "in the selection of countries, the design of the implementation, the interpretation, or the control of funding."

IMPACT OF AN EVALUATION

In the final presentation of the session, Carmela Green-Abate, the PEPFAR coordinator in Ethiopia, discussed how both the recent IOM PEPFAR evaluation and a prior IOM evaluation earlier in the implementation of PEPFAR have been used to affect the program. She first noted that the independence of the IOM as the evaluator allowed the evaluations to have a significant impact on the program, both in terms of funding and in a change in the program's emphasis from getting medication to those with HIV/AIDS to one of preventing infection in the first place. The need to make this change was highlighted in the first of the two evaluations, and the success in making this transformation was highlighted in the second. The first evaluation also pointed out the need to develop health system capacity, and this finding was reflected in increased funding for this type of activity in the second round of PEPFAR grants.

Green-Abate noted that the lack of country-specific findings in the evaluation was frustrating and limiting. "Going forward, I think that there are opportunities to document best practices in the evaluation," she said. She added, however, that based in part on the second evaluation, Congress has authorized a third phase of the program. "Without these independent evaluations, I do not think that Congress would have continued to fund this program at the same level," she said.

She also remarked that the second evaluation emphasized knowledge management, including monitoring evaluation, innovation, and research. This has contributed to a new monitoring and evaluation framework from PEPFAR that is still being rolled out, but an enormous dilemma at the country level is alignment with the countries and the speed of the roll out. "If you really do want country ownership, you need to have time in which countries can change their health management and information systems in line and not have different systems."

In closing, Green-Abate said that there is a real need to build capacity and involve more Africans in the program. "If you look at the trials, they are not led by Africans, and PEPFAR does not support their participation at scientific meetings. How can you expect country-level capacity to increase?" she asked. "I would suggest that the U.S. government is in a unique position to move forward in the third phase of PEPFAR to support the opportunities for innovative research and evaluation at the regional or country level in Africa." In response to a question about what could be done to build more capacity in Africa, Green-Abate cited the Medical Education Partnership Initiative, a $10 million program funded by PEPFAR, as one approach that may work. This program designates African institutions and universities as the principal investigators, with U.S. universities serving as subcontractors. Its strength, said Green-Abate, is that it does not take talented African researchers out of their institutions and bring them to the United States, but rather leaves those excellent investigators in place where they can nurture younger investigators. "I think initiatives in which the African academic institutions are in charge, with links to the rest of the world, offer a real opportunity," she said. During further discussion about building capacity,

Christopher Whitty from DFID added that in his opinion there is a real need to build up African institutions, but that "there are already African scientists who should be able to be at the forefront of doing this kind of work." However, he said that while his organization often receives grant applications that list African investigators, he is frequently disappointed when the publication comes out and there are no African authors. Whitty described it as shameful when American co-investigators do not sufficiently involve their African colleagues once a grant is secured.

OTHER TOPICS RAISED IN DISCUSSION

Sangeeta Mookherji of George Washington University, asked how the field can ensure that there is independence and objectivity when it comes to analyzing and interpreting data, not just collecting data. Black cited the PEPFAR evaluation as an example where the interpretation and analysis of data was independent, even though some of the data came from the program itself. The extensive review by outside experts helped ensure this independence. He also noted that there may be cases where program staff can provide insights that the evaluators can then respond to in their analysis, and he cited the evaluation of the PMI as an example of where program staff had a chance to comment on the analysis.

Whitty added while independence is critical to being able to trust an evaluation's results, it may be difficult to understand all of the details of a complex project without input from the people on the ground. The trade-off between independence and understanding is difficult, but achieving the right balance is critical. "If you go too far in either direction, you are going to fail," said Whitty. Lori Heise, from the London School of Hygiene and Tropical Medicine, asked if independence at the beginning of smaller projects might not be counterproductive. "I would argue, at the early stages of developing novel interventions, to have less independence between researchers and evaluators so that you are actually refining the program, and treat evaluation as a partnership."

Sanjeev Sridharan, University of Toronto, asked the panelists if they had any ideas about how to deal with evaluation timelines with large, complex programs. Rugg noted the importance of developing a plan of how to feed information to evaluators in a timely and frequent manner that can enable evaluations throughout the life of a program. "If you do that, I think then it is more palatable and [will meet] the needs of multiple information requesters." Whitty suggested evaluating subcomponents or particular questions within a much larger scheme. "Often, when you do that, you can, within the timeline you have, plan ahead, because most complex interventions have multiple interventions that are brought at different times in different places, and they allow certain subquestions to be answered quite well within the timelines, even if you do not have the luxury of being able to plan it right from the beginning and evaluate the whole thing as a package," he said.

Several of the presenters discussed the challenges of large evaluations that take place over multiple years and suggested different ways to evaluate or assess specific components of large-scale initiatives in a shorter time-frame to provide feedback more quickly. Green-Abate made a distinction between monitoring and evaluating. "Monitoring for me is something that we can report very quickly and we can get results," she said, noting that she believes that PEPFAR did an extraordinarily good job of this. While monitoring was target oriented and not designed to measure impact, "in every year we could actually say exactly what had been done and how many people had been reached." Evaluation, she said, is a high-level activity with a different purpose. Rugg cautioned that program monitoring data are important, but that "you have to know why you collect every single piece of information." A lot of the information that PEPFAR has in its huge databases is not used for program management decision making, she noted, "and therefore I think the program is hard pressed to show the value added from the money that goes into that program monitoring." Black added that, "I would say almost any program that is worth doing is worth evaluating or monitoring. I do respect there are differences. Getting information to improve the program is important for any program." Evaluation, he noted, does not always have to be about mortality impact or health outcome.

In response to a question from Sir George Alleyne, chancellor of the University of the West Indies and a member of the workshop planning committee, about whether all programs were evaluable, Rugg said that programs such as the UN Development Programme or WHO are evaluated not for the purpose of determining whether they should continue but to make them better, which is a different type of evaluation. Whitty said that evaluability is not a yes/no proposition but a spectrum that ranges from the obvious to the impossible. "Where you put the cutoff will depend on your resources and the importance of the question [you are trying to answer]," he said. "There are some things that are easily evaluable but probably not worth evaluating largely because they are not going to be done again."

4

Developing the Evaluation Design and Selecting Methods

Important Points Made by the Speakers

- Evaluations of complex initiatives require trade-offs in developing the evaluation design and choosing the methods.
- Evaluations of complex initiatives are well served by the use of a logic model, theory of change, results chain, impact pathway, or other framework to describe how the program is intended to create change and to identify potential unintended results.
- It is important to design the evaluation and interpret findings in the context of the environments in which initiatives are implemented and in the context of interrelated activities both within the same initiative and carried about by other stakeholders.
- Building measurement into the management of programming can be a powerful way of tracking causation.
- Standardization of data collection and analysis when feasible can improve comparability within and across evaluations.
- Despite guidance and resources that are available, many complex evaluations still fail to follow good practices.

Designing an evaluation involves many challenges and trade-offs. The members of the workshop's second panel discussed designing evaluations to understand not only whether an effect was achieved but also how and why. They also spoke of the importance of strategically thinking through different options for data collection and analysis methods and how those methods can be matched to the aims and questions of an evaluation, the available data, and the feasibility of implementing the methods with appropriate rigor. Finally, the panelists addressed ways of recognizing, understanding, and grappling with the complexity of an initiative being evaluated and of the contexts in which an initiative is implemented.

INSTITUTE OF MEDICINE EVALUATION OF PEPFAR

As was mentioned during the first panel, Congress has twice mandated that the IOM conduct an independent, external evaluation of the effects of PEPFAR. Deborah Rugg, a member of the IOM committee for the second independent evaluation of PEPFAR, explained that this most recent evaluation attempted to assess PEPFAR's contribution to the HIV response in partner countries and globally since the inception of the initiative in 2003. Thus, the task for the IOM was to design and then conduct an impact evaluation of a complex dynamic initiative with a wide range of supported activities and a global reach. The resulting evaluation was conducted over 4 years with an extensive planning phase followed by an intensive implementation phase. The evaluation was carried out by a volunteer expert committee for each phase, along with IOM staff and consultants with relevant expertise. The evaluation was comprehensive in terms of the overall program, but it was not an evaluation of country-specific programs, specific partners, or specific agencies. Rugg noted that the evaluation relied on a framework of contribution to impact rather than attribution.

A critical part of the early evaluation planning process was to carry out an evaluability assessment, which included the interpretation of the congressional mandate, the development of evaluation questions, and a mapping exercise to determine what data were available globally at the headquarters level and in the countries. As another critical and parallel part of the early planning process, the committee also explored the feasibility of various designs and methods that the IOM might use in its evaluation, ultimately deciding on a conceptual framework and developing a program impact pathway (see Figure 4-1). "This conceptual framework was then simplified in order to cover the diversity of programs, to communicate to a variety of audiences, and to be something that all of the technical areas could use to organize the committee's activity," explained Rugg.

The conceptual framework included the various inputs into the PEPFAR initiative, such as the considerable financial and technical assistance resources going into the PEPFAR initiative as well as the strategies, guidance, and planning activities that were significant in developing and implementing the initiative. Rugg noted that the committee also viewed PEPFAR's use of the evolving scientific evidence base as an input. In devel-

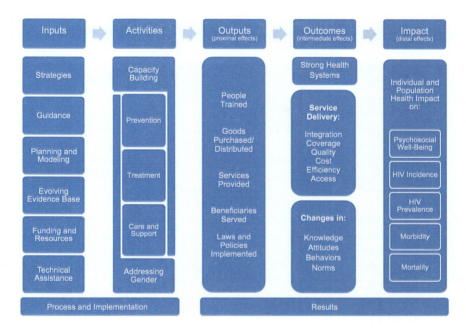

FIGURE 4-1 The program impact pathway for the Institute of Medicine's Second Evaluation of PEPFAR (2009–2013), as presented by Rugg.
SOURCE: IOM, 2013.

oping this framework, the IOM committee examined PEPFAR's capacity-building activities; the three areas of prevention, treatment, and care and support; and efforts to address gender equality in the initiative. The committee then looked at basic outcomes and tried to understand the impacts of PEPFAR in terms of proximal, intermediate, and distal effects.

"The outputs that we considered to be primary were outputs such as people trained, goods purchased and distributed, services provided, beneficiaries served, and the laws and policies that were designed and implemented," said Rugg. She explained that the basic outcomes for the evaluation were in the areas of strengthening health systems; specific service delivery areas focusing on the integration of services and the coverage, quality, cost, efficiency, and access to services; and looking at any resulting changes in knowledge, attitude, behavior, and norms of the beneficiaries as well as providers. Seeking to respond to the congressional mandate, the IOM committee focused on key impact areas that would allow it to comment on individual and population health impact, including psychosocial well-being, HIV incidence, HIV prevalence, morbidity, and mortality.

The end result was a hybrid evaluation design that was retrospective and cross-sectional in nature and included time trend data and time series analyses. This design had different in-depth approaches and different topical areas, which Rugg characterized as a nested design. It also used a mixed methods approach. "This mixed methods approach included complementary data from different data sources and used both qualitative and quantitative data in order to balance the limitations of each other," she said. The quality and rigor of the causal contribution analysis were improved through a triangulation approach among the different types of data and different analyses. When combined with the program impact pathway, this design provided a solid basis to help determine not just whether PEPFAR was affecting health outcomes but how and why.

In reflecting on the basic design, Rugg said that the value of a "whole of initiative" approach was that its findings could be interpreted in the context of the obvious interrelatedness of all the different activities conducted by PEPFAR. "We have long since moved beyond a time when interventions are isolated and single interventions have the effect we seek," said Rugg. "They are necessarily interrelated and interdependent."

The trade-offs associated with this design were the necessary duration of the evaluation and the limited data collection and depth of analysis in any one area of activity. "We could not drill down because of our focus at the higher, whole initiative level," she explained. The "whole of initiative" approach also meant trade-offs in evaluation use in terms of the lack of country-specific findings described previously in Chapter 3, but she noted that the candor achieved by not identifying countries was critical to the quality and credibility of the data.

Rugg closed her comments by offering some advice for future evaluation options of this now mature initiative. Rather than conducting a single periodic evaluation to assess the impact of the entire initiative, it might be more strategic to create a portfolio of external evaluations, with each evaluation focused on a more narrow, high-priority, complex area of the initiative (e.g., interventions to increase women's access to services or activities to strengthen public health laboratories) that could be completed in a shorter time frame. In addition, she advised that dissemination activities for these hypothetical evaluations focus on specific interpretations and applications of messages that could be tailored to specific countries, providing an opportunity for dialog without compromising the evaluation design in a way that would sacrifice candor and credibility.

GLOBAL FUND EVALUATION

Why is evaluating impact important to the Global Fund? Daniel Low-Beer, head of impact, results, and evaluation at the Global Fund, explained that the core purpose of the Global Fund is to achieve a sustainable and significant contribution to the reduction of infections, illness, and death. To realize this goal, it has developed a new strategy of investing specifically for impact in terms of lives saved, infections averted, and meeting the Millennium Development Goals of reducing child mortality, improving maternal health, and combating HIV/AIDS, malaria, and tuberculosis. Today, a key part of the Global Fund's programming is to invest more strategically for impact and to promote prioritization through its management focus.

The definitions of impact that the Global Fund uses for its evaluation have two components: assessing final disease outcomes and impact, and assessing contribution and causation along the results chain. For the first component at the epidemiological stage, Low-Beer explained, the evaluation looks at two primary questions. The first asks if there has been a change in disease mortality and morbidity or incidence and prevalence and if that change has been positive or negative. The second asks if there has been a change in outcomes, positive or negative. In terms of the second component of impact, contribution and causation, the evaluation asks if interventions, as well as other competing explanations such as deforestation and climate change, contributed to and resulted in these impacts, both positive and negative. To enable the evaluation of impact, the Global Fund has established a $10 million fund for investing in data infrastructures in target countries to enable rigorous analysis; disaggregation of data by time, person, and place; and inclusion of comparison groups where feasible.

Low-Beer said that the Global Fund's technical committee is seeking to establish an independent yet practical approach to evaluation that can be integrated into the way the Global Fund makes grants and develops policies. Its approach to impact reviews is to:

- involve partners and build on in-country evaluation programs;
- make the evaluations periodic so they occur at regular intervals coordinated with in-country evaluations;
- use a plausibility design to provide evidence of impact, both positive and negative impact, and taking into account nonprogram influences;
- build country platforms that build on national systems and includes program reviews; and
- produce practical results and recommendations for grant management, grant renewal, and reprogramming.

In essence, said Low-Beer, the Global Fund has shifted its focus and funding away from a single overarching evaluation once every 5 years, to investing in a more continuous form of evaluation—"from a 5-year evaluation to this challenge of 5 years of rolling evaluations." By the end of 2013, all key components of this new strategy were operational, and the Global Fund is now supporting 21 in-country program reviews that are part of its new funding model. Four thematic reviews on cross-cutting areas have been launched along with 17 data quality assessments that were agreed to by its partners and general managers in 10 countries. At the time of the workshop, the Global Fund's new funding model had been launched in Myanmar and Zimbabwe, and both Cambodia and Thailand have developed refocused national strategies. Some of the thematic reviews had already led to new grants, said Low-Beer, including a regional grant to evaluate artemisinin resistance that was based on one of the evaluations by the technical evaluations group. According to Low-Beer, a key issue is to determine the best way to use country program reviews to develop better programming and to improve grant making.

Low-Beer then described two examples to illustrate why it is important to establish impact up front in the Global Fund's programming. The first involved HIV prevention in Thailand, where the grant had been achieving many of its programmatic targets. "But when we looked at epidemiological trends, we saw high levels of HIV among injection drug users, increasing levels among men who have sex with men and male sex workers, and stable but not decreasing levels in female sex workers," said Low-Beer. These data show that while programmatic performance was good, impact was limited. Further review of the data suggested that it should be possible to increase coverage by focusing on the 27 provinces that accounted for 70 percent of new HIV infections, to use a network approach to deliver the packaged services to those who are most at risk, and to use innovative and robust monitoring approaches to support the delivery of HIV prevention services.

In Cambodia, the Global Fund put its HIV, tuberculosis, and malaria reviews together to identify common components of value. These reviews found that malaria deaths dropped by 80 percent and that this drop was linked to specific investments in the Global Fund's portfolio, such as the $5 million to $10 million spent on community workers and the scale-up of treatments and bed net use; in addition, there was a 45 percent decline in tuberculosis prevalence related to Global Fund grants. However, noted Low-Beer, the review found that HIV prevention efforts were stagnant despite successful high coverage of antiretroviral therapy.

One of the strengths of this approach is that it builds measurement into management of programming and the way the Global Fund invests in its grants. "The causative framework that relies on time, person, and place has been quite powerful," said Low-Beer. One of the current drawbacks of this approach is the variability in the quality of the program reviews, an issue that will take 2–3 years and investments by the Global Fund to address. This approach also requires strong political backing, both at the country and Global Fund level, to turn recommendations for national programs into grants that focus on impact. Low-Beer added that this approach works well only in countries where additional investments are made in country evaluation agendas and where there are trials, studies, and operational research. He also noted that these reviews use a series of questions that have been defined by a technical evaluation group and that start with impacts and outcomes. The reviews include funding for an independent consultant to ensure they are run independently.

AFFORDABLE MEDICINES FACILITY–MALARIA ASSESSMENT

The Affordable Medicines Facility–malaria (AMFm) was established to address problems with access to artemisinin-based combination therapies (ACTs) for malaria, the highly effective and recommended treatment for this disease. Catherine Goodman, senior lecturer in health economics and policy in the Department of Global Health and Development at the London School of Hygiene and Tropical Medicine, explained that, despite free or highly subsidized public-sector availability of ACTs, access through the public sector remains poor. As a result, many customers use less effective antimalarials or use artemisinin as a single agent, which could exacerbate the development of artemisinin resistance. To address these problems, the Global Fund created AMFm with the twin goals of contributing to malaria mortality reduction and delaying the development of artemisinin resistance by increasing the availability, affordability, market share, and use of quality-assured ACTs.

AMFm comprises three elements, said Goodman. First, the program negotiates with ACT manufacturers to reduce drug costs in both the public and private sectors. Second, the program provides a large buyer subsidy at the top of the global supply chain. Third, the program supports a range of in-country interventions to ensure effective scale up. AMFm was first implemented as eight national-scale pilot programs that enabled the participating countries to purchase ACTs from approved manufacturers at the subsidized, negotiated price. Within each country, the drugs were distributed through the standard public- or private-sector distribution chain, which means that the program has no control over where the drugs go within a given country.

Turning to the design of the AMFm evaluation, Goodman noted that because the intervention occurs on a national scale, control areas within the country were not possible. Instead, the evaluation relied on a pre- and post-test design with baseline and endpoint assessments. The key primary source of data was outlet surveys, which she explained are nationally representative surveys conducted at baseline and endline. The baseline surveys took place before the intervention began. The endline, which varied by country, was 6 to 15 months after the first subsidized drugs had arrived in the country. She and her colleagues surveyed all outlets that could possibly supply antimalarials. "We are looking at total market approach in the evaluation," said Goodman. Outlets included public and private health facilities, pharmacies and drug stores, general stores that stock antimalarials, or community health workers or vendors. "Whoever had antimalarials, we visited them."

To measure ACT availability, price, and market share, the survey used a cluster sampling approach stratified by urban and rural areas; it also used a sample size calculation based on detecting a 20 percentage point change in quality-assured ACT availability. For data on use of ACTs, the evaluators required household survey information, but as Goodman explains, "It was decided not to fund specific household surveys for this study ... largely due to cost considerations." Use of ACTs was certainly considered an important outcome, but several ongoing household surveys collect data on fever treatment, and the evaluation team hoped to use the data from these surveys. In the end, she added, the evaluation only had appropriately timed data from those types of surveys for five of the eight pilots. "The use data was somewhat incomplete," she said.

The next component of the evaluation design relied on the availability of careful documentation of the process of AMFm implementation and the context of the implementation in specific countries, such as the exact settings of the implementation and other activities that were occurring at the time of implementation. The evaluation also included a few extra studies, including one that looked specifically at distribution and use in remote areas of Ghana and Kenya and the role of the AMFm logo.

Goodman noted that once the evaluation was in progress, the Global Fund Secretariat contracted with an independent group from the University of California, San Francisco, to develop recommendations for success metrics that would be reasonable to expect 1 year after the effective start date of AMFm (see Figure 4-2). "When we were doing the evaluation, what we were actually testing was not whether there had been a significant change over time but whether countries had significantly exceeded the success metric and whether we could be confident that they had met these targets," said Goodman.

Goodman then highlighted a number of strengths and limitations of the AMFm evaluation. One of the strengths was that the evaluation was conducted in all eight operational pilot projects, which represented a wide range of contexts. The primary outlet survey data were from nationally representative surveys and drew on well-developed methods being used by the ACTwatch monitoring program.[1] The evaluation also had careful standardization of data collection and analysis across the pilots, and although

---

[1] More information is available at http://www.actwatch.info (accessed April 10, 2014).

Objectiv	Success benchmark
Availability	1. **20 percentage point increase** from baseline to endline in the percentage of outlets stocking ALL quality assure ACTs (QAACTs) (both with and without the AMFm logo) among outlets stocking antimalarials
Price	2. Median price of one adult equivalent treatment dose (AETD) of AMFm QAACTs (with the logo) is **less than 3 times** the median price of one AETD of the most popular antimalarial in tablet form which is not a QAACT (in private for-profit outlets)
	3. Median price of one AETD of AMFm QAACTs (with the logo) is **less than** the median price of one AETD of oral artemisinin monotherapy (AMT) tablets (in private for-profit outlets)
Use	4. **5 percentage point increase** from baseline in percentage of children under age 5 years with fever in the last 2 weeks who received ACT treatment
Market share	5. Increase in market share of ALL QAACTS of **10 percentage points** from baseline to endline
	6. **Decrease** in market share of AMTs (all oral dosage forms) from baseline to endline

FIGURE 4-2 Success metrics for AMFm evaluation.
SOURCE: Goodman, 2014.

actual data collection was done by different agencies, not by the evaluation team, the evaluation team was involved in quality assurance throughout the data collection process. While there were no controls for this evaluation, the team was able to assess plausibility using the carefully documented information on process and context, and it was able to conduct its evaluation independently.

Regarding limitations of the evaluation, Goodman listed the short timeline for the evaluation between AMFm implementation and the endline outlet survey in some countries as a challenging issue, along with the need to rely on secondary household survey data to assess one of the key outcomes. While the evaluation did cover eight countries, that is still a limited number, so extrapolation to countries with different antimalarial markets needs to be done with caution. Also, a number of areas were beyond the scope of this evaluation, such as patient adherence to ACT, the prevalence of counterfeit drugs, and targeting by parasitemia status—that is, whether the patients receiving ACT actually had malaria.

One of the biggest concerns, said Goodman, was the fact that there were no comparators for the evaluation. One possible methodological solution was that, while it was not possible to create comparison areas within the pilot settings, it might have been possible to create comparison areas in other countries. The evaluation team debated this approach and concluded that the challenges of choosing comparison countries were too great for this evaluation. "There are so many big differences in context and in the implementation of other malaria control strategies," said Goodman. These differences between pilot AMFm countries and potential comparison countries raised important questions. "Are we trying to compare with the status quo in other countries? Are we trying to compare with other countries that have implemented other strategies, like community health workers, for instance? It is quite difficult to know how to go about those comparisons even if they were valid."

She noted, too, there is a selection bias in terms of meeting the criteria to be an AMFm pilot country and the challenge of finding additional comparison countries that matched those same criteria. There was also a concern about the potential flow of drugs across national borders and other ways in which the AMFm pilot in some countries might have led to effects in other nonpilot countries—as well as the fact that AMFm may have had a role in shaping the global market for relatively low-cost ACTs, which could have influenced the market as a whole and the cost of production. "One cannot be absolutely sure what the counterfactual results would have been in the absence of AMFm," she noted. Finally, collecting sufficient comparator data in other countries would have been costly.

THE SEARCH FOR GOOD PRACTICE IN COMPLEX EVALUATIONS

In the final presentation of this panel, Elliot Stern, emeritus professor of evaluation research at Lancaster University and visiting professor at Bristol University, discussed some of the lessons he has learned about good practices in evaluation design during his career and his experiences reviewing evaluations, sitting on quality assurance bodies, and helping to draw up terms of reference. He said, "What is amazing, despite all the guidance and debates and conferences like this and the investments that have taken place, is how difficult it is in truly complex areas to find good practice." For example, even in major evaluations commissioned by major bodies, evaluation questions can be absent or poorly formulated, context is often ignored, and there is poor use of theory even when there is an acknowledged need for explanations of how and why. Other shortcomings that he noted include poor stakeholder engagement, which is often associated with weak construct validity; the continued application of Humean designs that look for the single cause of a single effect even after recognizing that there are multiple causes with multiple effects; weaknesses in the bases for causal claims; and poor integration of multiple methods.

To illustrate the challenges of finding good practices for evaluating complex programs, Stern discussed evaluations of the Consultative Group on International Agricultural Research (CGIAR) Natural Resource Management Research (NRM-R) programs, and in particular, the Research Program on Aquatic Agricultural Systems being run in the Lake Victoria area, the Mekong Delta, and the Coral Triangle. The NRM-R, explained Stern, runs multileveled, multilocation interventions operating at the farm, landscape, regional, and global levels. It combines participatory and technological interventions in ways designed to change the behavior of individuals, households, institutions, and markets, as well as to change policies. NRM-R deploys research and local tacit knowledge through action research, and it engages policy makers, scientists, and community partners to collaboratively plan for change that will in the end strengthen natural resource management in the target region.

Looking at the goals of the Research Program on Aquatic Agricultural Systems, Stern characterized them as generic and difficult to pin down. "We are talking about sustainable productivity gains for system-dependent households, improved markets and services for the poor and vulnerable, strengthened resilience and adaptive capacity, reduced gender disparities in access to and control of resources and decision making, and improvements in policy and institutions to support pro-poor, gender-equitable, and sustainable development," he said. Evaluating outcomes for these goals is challenging without reducing them to specific activities, but doing so "involves a trade-off between being able to say something about the program as opposed to being able to say something about a particular scheme in a particular area," said Stern.

One of the building blocks of a successful evaluation is developing an adequate theory of change. Doing so requires identifying the critical links in program planning, implementation, and delivery and identifying critical conditions, assumptions, and supporting factors. It is also necessary to identify rivals to the "official" program theory, not simply develop an evaluation that has what Stern called a "confirmatory bias" resulting from a design that evaluates a program from the perspective of how it is supposed to work rather than how a program actually is working. Another component of an adequate theory of change is a means of assessing the contexts of program implementation. In terms of causality, it is important to remember that most programs do not cause results singlehandedly; rather, they make a difference or contribute to results. Rarely, said Stern, is a program both necessary and sufficient by itself to produce positive results without other supporting factors. Using fish farming as an example, the initiative components could include start-up funding, provision of fingerlings, low-cost fish food, and advice on improved fish farming techniques. Supporting factors could be an adequate number of farmers initially convinced to try fish farming and an adequate market for fish produced over and above a family's consumption. In this case, the initiative factors made a difference, but were more likely to do so if the supporting factors were also present.

The evaluation questions have important implications concerning design choices, yet too often evaluators place insufficient emphasis on how these questions are formulated, Stern said. Asking if an observed change can be attributed to the intervention requires a counterfactual design; asking how an intervention makes a difference is difficult to answer without theory; asking whether an intervention will work elsewhere requires some consideration of contexts and mechanisms.

The other major building block for developing a good evaluation design involves understanding the attributes of a program and designing in a way that will account for them. One of the attributes of the NRM-R program, for example, is that it recognizes that ecosystems mediate social and ecological systems. As a result, multidisciplinary knowledge and theory need to be used when designing an evaluation. In addition, the lack of market-based coordination of resource use by stakeholders means that an evaluation design will have to account for the likelihood of conflicts and will need methods to evaluate conflicts and collective action. The presence of level-specific effects in a multilevel program highlights the importance of nested designs that may require different theories and methods at each level, which creates the challenge of achieving vertical integration between levels. Uncertain and extended change trajectories, in which markets change rapidly but landscapes change over decades, requires the use of iterative rather than fixed designs accompanied by extended longitudinal modeling. Stern noted, too, that because systems integration involves trade-offs, the use of game theory and modeling may be needed to capture both trade-offs and holistic factors that might be having an impact.

"The key message that I have been trying to emphasize is not only that design is important, but if you want quality evaluations, you have to invest in it," Stern said in closing. "We suggest that up to 20 percent of the budget available for evaluation ought to be invested in good design work. That does not mean sitting and writing a proposal, but it does mean revisiting the design issues over time. The more complex the program, the more design matters—and it takes time. If you get the logic of description, explanation, and causal inference right, methods follow more easily."

OTHER TOPICS RAISED IN DISCUSSION

To start the discussion, moderator and workshop planning committee member Kara Hanson, who is professor of health system economics at the London School of Hygiene and Tropical Medicine, asked the panelists to speak briefly about (1) how they conceived of context in designing their evaluation and (2) the methodological approaches that exist to understand the effects of context, particularly for complex interventions. Goodman replied that she and her colleagues tried to collect data on context within each of the countries being studied. "For instance, what is the antimalarial market like in a given country and how has that affected how AMFm is rolled out," she said. "If there has been a change in one of the key outcomes, is there anything else that is plausibly responsible for this apart from AMFm? We tried to look at all of those things mainly through qualitative and some quantitative data toward the endline."

The Global Fund, said Low-Beer, takes an open approach to causation that considers alternative hypotheses involving context as opposed to looking just at whether an individual intervention produces an observed effect. In addition, he and his colleagues often start with impacts and outcomes and then work back along the causal chain to try to identify other hypotheses of change that could be dependent on context. Stern added, "There is an overall question of the object of evaluation, which defines the context. If you take a realist ontology where you are actually looking at mechanisms in context and being able to understand why things work in one place and not in another, that inevitably drives you toward trying to understand how is it that the context has made the difference. To some extent, the rediscovery of context can occur much later in the train of events. It can occur when you get to the stage that you have this puzzling data. And it may only be then that the nature of that context might be revealed."

In the PEPFAR evaluation, said Rugg, the issue of context came up in the early phases of the design. She explained that a conceptual model was developed that embedded the PEPFAR operations in the context of many other factors in each country. Then, in the implementation phase, the evaluators looked at a variety of indicators that were compared across countries to give a contextual background of the environment in which PEPFAR was operating. The significant qualitative data collection component also explored contextual issues in the countries that were visited. Rugg added that what is equally important but rarely considered concerning context is the influence of individuals and charismatic leaders on a program's success or failure.

In response to a question from Sangeeta Mookherji from George Washington University about whether the panelists were thinking about supporting factors as part of context, Hanson noted and Stern agreed that the field needs some clarification in the language to communicate such issues clearly. Stern added, "It is quite different to talk about nonprogram things and those things that we can influence and the much more causative specific contextual or supporting factors that might affect a particular change in a particular place."

A discussion about stakeholder involvement in planning and reviewing evaluations, prompted by a question from Carlo Carugi of the Global

Environment Facility, highlighted a variety of reasons why it may be useful to involve stakeholders at different stages of the evaluation process. Rugg noted that the PEPFAR evaluation team had opportunities to engage with staff from PEPFAR and Congress to understand the intent of the mandate, as well as to discuss the strategic plan for the evaluation after the publication of a planning phase report, when there was also an opportunity for public engagement. Bridget Kelly, one of the two IOM study co-directors for the evaluation, added that an operational planning phase included two pilot country visits, which in addition to being data collection trips were also an opportunity to elicit that kind of stakeholder understanding of how things operate in practice, to learn what kind of data requests would be feasible and timely, and to pilot tools for primary data collection.

Goodman said that the AMFm team held a meeting of the pilot countries after producing a first draft of their report to debate the results, and during this meeting at least some of the countries were, as she put it, "not feeling happy with the way the evaluation was framed for their country." She added that the international malaria community was brought in at the design stage as part of the advisory team that supported the development of the evaluation design.

Finally, in response to a question from Ruth Levine, director of the Global Development and Population Program at the William and Flora Hewlett Foundation Evaluations, about why evaluations break what she called "Evaluation 101 rules," Stern singled out overambitious and under-funded terms of reference for evaluations, poor governance, and insufficient experience on the part of those conducting evaluations.

5

Mapping Data Sources and Gathering and Assessing Data

Important Points Made by the Speakers

- When planning an evaluation, the feasibility of collecting the necessary data is an important consideration.
- Standardized data collection and analysis methods can help assure quality.
- The time frame and budget of an evaluation are critical factors in designing data collection and analysis for a complex evaluation.
- Routinely collected program data can be a rich and efficient source of information for program evaluation.
- Financial data can help assess the efficiency of a program and the return on an investment.
- A large-scale data infrastructure that includes a wide variety of data sources could be a powerful research tool.

The *sine qua non* of evaluation is data, but it is also the rock upon which many hopes are dashed for evaluators and evaluands. In this session, six panelists discussed the importance of and strategies for identifying and assessing potential data sources. At the beginning of the panel, session moderator and workshop planning committee member Ann Kurth, professor of nursing, medicine, and public health at New York University, noted the importance of data both for the design and for the execution of an evaluation. Data issues include the kinds of data needed across program components, the availability of data, metrics, the disaggregation of data, routinely collected versus new data, who owns the data, what format the data are in, and what mechanisms are used to share data. In addition, questions about data quality can arise, particularly when data are being collected by people outside of the evaluation team. A major decision point in the process of designing an evaluation is determining the feasibility of collecting and accessing all necessary data.

DATA MAPPING IN THE IOM EVALUATION OF PEPFAR

Kurth, who was also a member of the IOM committee for the evaluation of PEPFAR, went on to describe how, in designing the evaluation, the team mapped available data sources as well as those that might need to be collected against the evaluation's goals and questions (IOM, 2013). The objective of the data mapping was to identify complementary data sources to address the evaluation questions using the program impact framework of inputs, activities, outputs, outcomes, and impact. In each of these levels of the framework, and in each of the technical areas evaluated, questions germane to the evaluation were developed. Data sources for answering the questions then were identified, whether monitoring, financial, surveillance, interview, document review, or other types of data. Where data were not available or ideal, the feasibility of getting the necessary data was assessed.

This mapping process took into account the priority of the questions to be answered, said Kurth. Not all questions could be answered given the project's time frame, geographic scope, and data availability. Also, some data were available only for certain time periods or subsets of the program. The initial data mapping was driven by the need to understand what data sources were actually available and developed into an iterative process of matching data sources with evaluation questions and the data needed to answer them.

DATA ISSUES IN THE GLOBAL FUND EVALUATION

Workshop planning committee member Martin Vaessen, senior vice president at ICF International, discussed data issues involved in the Global Fund's evaluation of the impact of collective efforts in reducing the disease burden of HIV/AIDS, tuberculosis, and malaria in 18 countries. All 18 countries, he explained, had national data records on all three diseases, but an extensive set of new data was collected via surveys in 8 countries, with data collection concentrated at the district level within a country. The evaluators did have a problem at the district level in that they wanted to classify districts as high performing or low performing but found it difficult to get all of the district-level information that would enable that type of classification. As a result, district classification was not used for the analysis.

Vaessen commented that these data were not collected by the evaluators or even by the Global Fund but by local organizations with assistance from individuals tasked with carrying out the evaluation. The data collection effort was "a lot of work" and very difficult, said Vaessen. It was a challenge to go to each district in a country and figure out how many health facilities were operating, how many nongovernmental organizations (NGOs) were working in the district, and how many civil society organizations were providing particular services to HIV/AIDS patients. He emphasized this point because part of the data mapping exercise that should be done in planning an evaluation also has to include feasibility—is it really doable to collect the necessary data? "We need to define who it is that will actually access those sources and get that information," said Vaessen. "It is key that we have strong local implementing agencies that we can work with, that listen to the people, that are working with them in terms of providing technical assistance, and that are open to working according to the guidelines established for the evaluation. This is not always the case." In the case of the Global Fund evaluation, three countries dropped out because they did not want to participate in data collection. "Those are the realities we have to deal with," Vaessen said.

Overall, the household surveys and facility surveys provided data that were of reasonable or good quality, but for most other information data quality was uneven across countries. For example, good financial information was almost impossible to obtain. One issue that arose was the need to pre-test some of the surveys in one country before expanding data collection to all the countries, an activity for which there was not always time given the timeline for the evaluation.

Based on his experience, Vaessen listed three steps that evaluators need to pay attention to when thinking about data collection. First, define all of the indicators that need to be measured. Preferably, he said, the indicators should be standardized and harmonized with other data collection efforts to avoid a proliferation of indicators that differ sometimes in a minor way but are not the same. Second, establish procedures for data collection, and decide on inclusion and exclusion of indicators. This step requires strengthening data collection systems based on an analysis of whether or not existing systems support the collection of good quality data. An evaluation or evaluation team may decide that "it may be too difficult or too cumbersome to collect certain indicators," said Vaessen. Finally, establish procedures to carry out frequent data quality assessments to ensure that the data are accurate, complete, and timely and that they can be aggregated and analyzed.

Vaessen noted there is a separate country report for each country participating in the Global Fund evaluation, and the richness of the information in the country reports is much greater than the synthesis report, which tried to draw general conclusions. These country reports contain more detailed information about data sources, completeness, and quality. This information is a contribution of the Global Fund that countries can use to improve data sources if they choose to do so.

DATA APPROACH AND CHALLENGES IN THE AFFORDABLE MEDICINES FACILITY–MALARIA EVALUATION

One of the strengths of the AMFm evaluation was the ability to use good quality assurance procedures with regard to the primary data, said Kara Hanson, professor of health system economics at the London School of Hygiene and Tropical Medicine. The AMFm team was able to start with methods that were developed by the ACTwatch monitoring program[1] for conducting outlet surveys, which included sampling techniques, the use of training materials, and analysis plans (Tougher et al., 2012). "We were able to develop for all eight pilots standardized questionnaires and a strong set of training materials and standard operating procedures for undertaking the outlet surveys," she explained. In addition, she added, "The team members participated in most of the training at baseline and at endline in all eight of the pilots."

The AMFm team also developed common data cleaning guidelines and analysis plans and gave responsibility for the analysis of the outlet survey data to the contractors who collected those data. The independent evaluation team then reviewed the results, performed the analysis of the changes over time between baseline and endline, and integrated the quantitative data with the qualitative country case study data to interpret and understand what was going on in each country.

In terms of challenges, the timing of the outlet surveys proved to be important. In Nigeria, for example, the time between baseline and when the first drugs arrived in country was 15 months, while in Kenya the time between baseline and the arrival of drugs was only 2 months. Hanson noted that while the longer time period in Nigeria could be a source of bias, "We were fairly certain that not a great deal was going on in terms of antimalarial drug supply in that intermittent period, particularly in the private sector." There were also significant differences across the eight countries between the arrival of the first co-paid drugs and the endline survey, as well as between scale-up of the information, education, and communication and behavior change communication efforts and the survey, with one country never implementing those efforts and two countries suspending them before

---

[1] More information is available at http://www.actwatch.info (accessed April 10, 2014).

the endline surveys were conducted. "What this raises is the challenge of trying to plan large-scale survey operations and the unpredictability of the start of an intervention when you are reliant on these complex processes," said Hanson.

Another challenge had to do with the availability and interpretation of household surveys. ACT use was one of the four outcomes that the AMFm evaluation was supposed to measure, but the collection of the primary household data was removed from the design even before the contract was issued because of cost, explained Hanson. The evaluation team knew that they were going to have to rely on existing surveys if the surveys fit the evaluation design time frame. Hanson noted that there was some ambivalence among AMFm stakeholders about whether use should even be evaluated given the short time frame between initiation of the program and the evaluation. In the end, the evaluation team relied on secondary data using some inclusion criteria. "We said that in order to be eligible as a baseline, a household survey had to be undertaken no more than 2 years before the beginning of the program and that the endline had to be at least 6 months after the arrival of the first co-paid drugs."

In the end, five countries had appropriately timed endline data, but unfortunately, neither Kenya nor Ghana, the two countries that were believed to be fast moving, strong implementers, had appropriately timed household survey data. In addition to the limited availability of endline data, Hanson noted that most of the surveys only measured ACT use among children and that there was limited control over the design of the survey and the training given to the interviewers. It was also difficult to predict when survey data were going to be available for analysis.

A third challenge was tied to the 2009 WHO recommendation that antimalarial drugs be given with a parasitological diagnosis, which led many countries to focus on expanding access to ACTs. That action, said Hanson, changed the discourse on the balance between access to ACTs and ensuring that the drugs are going to people with parasites. AMFm was launched at about the same time, which led to a primary indicator being changed during the course of the evaluation period. As a result, use results were difficult to interpret.

Summarizing the key lessons from the AMFm evaluation, Hanson said the team learned about the importance of standardizing data collection and analysis methods to assure quality. They also recognized the challenges of mounting a large primary data collection exercise that is constrained on one side by epidemiology and logistics and on the other side by being dependent on countries for data that may not be forthcoming on the necessary timeline. Finally, relying on secondary analysis for something that turned out to be a key outcome was a limitation, said Hanson. "In fact, the TERG report on the evaluation points out the absence of evidence on use. The pieces just do not all link up."

PRESIDENT'S MALARIA INITIATIVE EVALUATION

The PMI evaluation had five objectives, Jonathan Simon, Robert A. Knox Professor and director of the Center for Global Health and Development at Boston University, reminded the workshop:

1. Review management's use of resources and management quality.
2. Evaluate the program's practices for getting the technical package of interventions into the focused countries.
3. Evaluate the partner environment to determine if the PMI was in the right niche given the importance of other efforts such as those of the Global Fund.
4. Evaluate the PMI's impact.
5. Make recommendations, which was not a data-driven issue.

"Within those five objectives, we had a number of different nails that we had to hammer, and we used different approaches or techniques or different types of data for that," said Simon.

For the first objective, a qualitative management review exercise, the primary sources of data were key stakeholder interviews with those in PMI leadership positions, as well as global, regional, and in-country stakeholders who benefit from the initiative. This was a relatively straightforward activity, Simon explained, because the stakeholders had asked for the review and were readily accessible. For the second objective, which was to try to get at what the program was doing, the evaluators used a mixed methods approach because they needed to look both at quantitative data about the key interventions and at some qualitative data about strengthening health systems or capacity strengthening within national malaria control programs. Here, program-based data from the donors, particularly the Global Fund, were useful because they provided information on how many drugs were bought and how many mosquito nets were sent into a country, though they revealed nothing about distribution or consumption, said Simon. It was more difficult, he said, to get at the issue of whether the PMI was strengthening health systems or national malaria control efforts.

Impact evaluation was the core objective of the evaluation, and Simon acknowledged that the 5 countries in which the evaluation team did in-depth studies were picked in part because they had better data than did the other 10 countries, where better data was defined as at least two and in some cases three data points on change in all-cause child mortality. "We did not have a direct measure of malaria-associated deaths averted, so we used the all-cause child mortality as a proxy for that, malaria being a big part of that pattern of death," Simon noted.

Much like the AMFm evaluation team, the PMI evaluation team was able to use data from other sources, such as the Demographic and Health Surveys (DHS), for primary and secondary data on all-cause mortality reduction. "We know both the strengths and weaknesses of those data and how they are constructed," explained Simon. Access to those data, he added, was not a problem. What was an issue was the quality of the data obtained from the in-country information systems and access to those data. In addition, little data analysis had occurred in many countries, yet those nations were reluctant to let the evaluation team analyze raw data. Access to raw data was also an issue with some of the larger philanthropies.

Simon concluded his remarks by situating the challenges of pursuing multiple sources of data as part of the complexity involved in conducting large-scale program evaluation on a short time frame and with a limited budget. "You are really in the realm of can you make a believable, plausible argument that associates the investments made by the global community and the national governments to minimize the impact of malaria to the activities that we were able to show did occur in terms of commodity, in terms of training, in terms of accessibility at health systems," said Simon. "It is a leap of faith. A lot of this evaluation requires a healthy skepticism, and then at the end of the day everybody decides just how far of a leap are they willing to make."

USING ROUTINE PROGRAM DATA

Drawing on the experience of the International Center for AIDS Care and Treatment (ICAP) as a large PEPFAR implementing partner supporting the scale-up of HIV services in approximately 20 countries over the past 8 years, Batya Elul, assistant professor of clinical epidemiology at Columbia University's Mailman School of Public Health, spoke about the nuts and bolts of using routinely collected data and publically available data for program evaluation. In many of its evaluations and research studies on the delivery of HIV/AIDS services, ICAP regularly uses four data sources:

1. Aggregate indicator data collected quarterly from 1.6 million patients at more than 3,000 facilities
2. De-identified clinical data collected quarterly with institutional review board (IRB) approval from 960,000 patients at 311 facilities
3. Annual clinical survey data from 1,017 care and treatment clinics and 730 laboratories

4. Community-level data from between 50 and 75 regions that are
    mapped at the subnational level to the regions in which health
    facilities that ICAP supports are located.

With these data in mind, ICAP's evaluation framework seeks to assess
the variation in key HIV care and treatment program outcomes by site
and determine the extent to which facility- and community-level factors
are associated with outcome, Elul explained. This framework recognizes
there is a substantial variation in the way HIV programs are scaled up both
within and between countries and takes advantage of this natural variation to identify which approaches are optimal by using largely hierarchical
modeling. Elul noted that, as is commonly the case when using routinely
collected data, ICAP has to contend with data quality issues. It addresses
these issues by conducting data quality assurance at the facility level, by
checking for completeness and consistency, through automated checks into
a web-based reporting and management system, and at the analytical stage.

As an example of the challenges inherent in working with this type
of data, Elul cited an evaluation of how many patients on antiretroviral
therapy were retained over time. This evaluation used data from three
implementing partners in a single country. Data from one partner showed
that they retained all of their patients, data from a second partner showed
essentially no retention, and the third had great fluctuations from 100
percent to no retention over time. Elul noted that they are still determining
whether this is a data quality issue or reality, but this is difficult because
many of the sites are small, with cohorts as small as five patients. After discussions with the implementing partners, it was decided to remove specific
data points only if the partners could provide very detailed documentation
and justifiable documentation as to why these values could be considered
poor data quality.

Even when implementing partners work hard to ensure data quality,
monitoring and evaluation systems are often not set up to facilitate analysis.
To ensure that data are accessible for analysis, ICAP uses unique site codes,
geocoding of sites, and data dictionaries, and it built its monitoring and
evaluation system to easily export a standardized analytic file along with
a standardized data dictionary to minimize the need for data managers or
programmers to create analysis files. To address potentially problematic
issues involving data ownership, ICAP has established principles of collaboration with each host government for its evaluation framework. These
principles include IRB approvals, the scope of the analyses, and the use of
data in multicountry analyses.

In conclusion, Elul stated, "Despite all the challenges of using routinely
collected program data, particularly when combined with publicly available
data, they are rich, highly underutilized, and often the most generalizable

and efficient source of information for program evaluation. When merged together, these data become much more powerful and lend themselves to multilevel analyses." That said, she added that it is essential to assess data quality at all phases of program evaluation or monitoring and that implementing partners need to do more to ensure their monitoring and evaluation systems facilitate data use for analysis.

WORKING WITH FINANCIAL DATA

As had been discussed previously, all data must be fit for purpose, and the purpose of financial data differs from that of programmatic data, said Victoria Fan, research fellow at the Center for Global Development. "While programmatic data is used to assess the effectiveness of activities, financial data helps us to assess the efficiency and the value for money of our investments. It provides a crucial denominator of just how much value or good was achieved for every pound, pula, or peso." The goal of the Center for Global Development's More Health for the Money evaluation was to examine the value of various global health funding agencies, with a focus on the Global Fund and its key partners. The evaluation looked at four main domains: resource allocation, contracts, cost and spending, and performance verification.

While there are many types of financial data, Fan focused on two types: budgets or planned expenditures, and actual expenditures and costs. She noted that data access and availability can be a serious challenge. In their review of Global Fund data, Fan and her colleagues found that out of approximately 20 countries that were the highest recipients of HIV/AIDS funding, 40 percent of the grants did not reveal any budget information in their country grant agreements. Of those that did, data availability and accessibility varied greatly. "We really had very little sense of where funding was going," she said. In response, the Global Fund said that the data were available but not publicly accessible. "We argued that having such information publicly accessible was crucial for value for money given the large number of actors in this space," said Fan.

Turning to the subject of actual expenditures and costs, she remarked, "The Global Fund should be commended for its groundbreaking price and quality reporting system, which reveals the prices and quantities of six main drugs and commodities." To secure future funding, countries must report the prices that they obtained for their drugs to the Global Fund's data system. But while the Global Fund has done a good job with price and quality reporting, Fan believes the organization needs to do more work on measuring unit costs. "Collecting such data and unit costs is not easy, and it involves facility surveys and multiple types of checks," she said. As a counterexample, Fan observed that recently PEPFAR has done a terrific job of collecting and using data on unit costs. In a pilot program in Mozambique, for example, PEPFAR was able to use such data to drive a reduction in the range of unit costs as well as in the average unit cost paid in the country.

DEVELOPING A LARGE-SCALE DATA INFRASTRUCTURE

For the past decade, Peter Elias, a labor economist in the Institute for Employment Research at the University of Warwick, has devoted his time to developing a large-scale data infrastructure to support research efforts in the United Kingdom. This data structure has enabled researchers to assemble the world's largest household panel study, the world's largest birth cohort study, and, most recently, a mechanism that will enable a link between a variety of administrative datasets and the United Kingdom's national health survey data. In his presentation, he focused on an effort he carried out with the support of the Organisation for Economic Co-operation and Development (OECD) to take a science-driven approach to advance a global social science data agenda. This effort focused on digital data that were perhaps not designed for research but that would have research value if they could be made available, discoverable, useable, and fit for purpose. Such data include census data, administrative records, and records of transactions.

Elias listed several reasons for engaging in this effort, including enabling comparative work, providing the ability to consolidate data to study rare groups, and enlarging studies beyond national boundaries. Issues that need to be addressed include increasing the discoverability of data, using new forms of data such as Google Flu Trends or data mined from store loyalty cards, and developing new methods of collecting data that are more cost-effective than traditional survey methods. He noted that using new forms of data collected from the Internet or transaction histories raises ethical data access issues and it's important to consider whether or not people have given their consent for the data collected about them to be used for additional research. Elias remarked on the potential challenges of consent in this context. He noted that, for example, the European Union is considering a law that would require all researchers to seek consent for all research, which for these new kinds of digital data not designed for research would be both costly and lead to strongly biased results. Nonetheless, he acknowledged that when a law is being written across 27 countries, there must be "some underlying public dissatisfaction with the way in which we, as researchers, are using data at the moment, and we have to address that issue." Along those lines, it is important that the community address the issue of data security and data governance.

Another consideration is data compatibility across nations. "There are plenty of international classifications out there that we should use but that so often are not used," said Elias. "We ought to have ways in which we can collaborate to define what it is we are studying in ways that will enable us to share that information." Equally important are having good metadata that describe how data were provided and collected and the means to preserve data and metadata on a sustainable basis. "We are beginning to wake up to the fact that a lot of our data preservation and management systems are inadequate for the modern age with the deluge of data that is now upon us," stated Elias. He noted that many efforts are under way to address these issues. For example, the European Union funds the Council of European Social Science Data Archives that is now working to integrate large data archives in many countries.

In a report to OECD, Elias and his colleagues recommended that there needs to be more funding of research to explore the potential of new forms of data and more cooperation between official statistical providers and research communities. "In some countries, that hardly exists at all, which is quite incredible," said Elias. "We need to have better coordination of data management plans so that we know more about data before they are created, ... and we need to ensure that the international organizations are more connected." More incentives for international data sharing are also needed, Elias remarked, as are ways in which people who take responsibility for the development of these resources are professionally rewarded for their efforts, given that few of these efforts produce publications.

In response to a question from Kristen Stelljes of the Hewlett Foundation about whether any of these efforts involve African nations, Elias said that South Africa has expressed a strong interest in joining the next stage of work. He acknowledged that it is often difficult for some of the poorer nations to join an effort that is largely being promoted by the wealthier nations of the world. It is not surprising that we end up with recommendations about data sharing that are doable for one group of countries "but remain absolutely out of reach for many other countries because of a lack of resources, a lack of knowledge, and a lack of expertise," he said. "That is a real problem that we have to address."

OTHER TOPICS RAISED IN DISCUSSION

Data access and availability were prominent topics in the discussion session. Elias pointed out that politics can be a powerful influence on data access. "At one point you will find there is great access and great cooperation, and then suddenly the barrier comes down and you cannot do something or you cannot publish something or you cannot take any data away or you cannot bring in people who you want to bring in.... It just hits a brick wall."

Simon pointed to four issues involved in data access. Having a strong relationship with investigators in a country can enable access that would not be the case with less strong relationships. "Level one is who do you know." Second, scientists tend to be more willing to share data than science managers, particularly governmental science managers. Third, some countries are more sensitive to sharing data than are others. Finally, some countries are more reluctant to share certain types of data, such as biological information, than other types. Vaessen added that writing provisions for data sharing into program agreements can avoid later problems.

Simon observed that universities are among the worst institutions in making data freely available. The open data movement is putting pressure on institutions to release data and research results within given time frames, and universities can support this movement, for example, through line items for data publication and archiving. "It is on the academic community to push harder on these issues."

Elias said that data archiving and accessibility are especially important with new forms of data, such as information gathered from online activities. Ethical issues as well as issues of reproducibility will surround these data types.

6

Applying Qualitative Methods to Evaluation on a Large Scale

Important Points Made by the Speakers

- The need for training and mentoring, ongoing reflection and reflexivity, collecting data to the point of saturation, and ensuring the accuracy of the data collection process are principles of qualitative methods that are particularly relevant for evaluating large-scale programs.
- Openness to listening and learning are instruments of discovery in qualitative research.
- Relationships within a data team are valuable when challenging each other or providing critiques of data interpretation.
- Delineating a program's sphere of control, sphere of influence, and sphere of interest is important in understanding a program's role as a change agent.
- Stories about exceptional results can provide insights into the factors contributing to those results.

The use of qualitative methods in evaluating large-scale initiatives can help evaluators understand not only whether something works but how and why it works. This subject was covered in several of the full-panel discussions, but one concurrent session aimed to take a deeper look at the use of qualitative methods for evaluation.

RIGOR AND CREDIBILITY IN QUALITATIVE DESIGN

In the concurrent session on qualitative methods, Sharon Knight, professor of health education in the College of Health and Human Performance at East Carolina University, used the PEPFAR evaluation as an example of how to ensure the qualitative aspects of a large-scale, complex evaluation are as rigorous and credible as possible. She noted that there is no consensus in the literature as to what makes a rigorous qualitative evaluation design but that a few concepts appear repeatedly, such as the need for training and mentoring for those on the evaluation team who are not familiar with qualitative methods; ongoing reflection and reflexivity throughout the data collection and analysis processes; the concept of saturation, or collecting data to the point of redundancy; and ensuring the accuracy of the data collection process.

Qualitative approaches are also called naturalistic inquiry, Knight said, because they are field-based, nonmanipulative, and noncontrolled. Qualitative researchers go into situations with a mindset of appreciating what is already there. "In fact, you want to make every effort not to change the environment, and certainly not the participants." Knight cautioned against a tendency to drift toward trying to explain qualitative data with quantitative language because of the desire to understand or signify something as important numerically. One example of this is the tendency to believe something is important because many people said it rather than one or a few who may have had a more nuanced viewpoint. One of the premises of qualitative research and evaluation is the appreciation of multiple views of reality and different perspectives. "Even if you have an *n* of one with a particular perspective that differs from everyone else's, that perspective deserves to be honored. It's not a situation where you have to throw it away because it's an outlier. Instead, you try to understand it, and certainly not ignore it," said Knight.

In a qualitative evaluation, she added, it is important to remember that the evaluator is an instrument of discovery that needs to listen, learn, and ask more. "Openness is a stance that we as evaluators should embrace," Knight stated, "and open-ended questions are the kind of questions we all strive for because it makes it more likely for the participant to be able to tell us the stories that really interest us." In the same vein, she said that everything is data in this kind of study, but that nothing becomes data unless it is documented and becomes part of the record. It is ethically important to ensure that each individual has given their consent before their words are captured or documented to be used as data. Knight added that in the PEPFAR evaluation, project leadership reinforced these ideas continually.

For the IOM's evaluation of PEPFAR, both staff and committee members were trained in qualitative methods. Formal training occurred in a 1-week workshop with the IOM staff on the evaluation team. "Team training," said Knight, "has to begin with thinking about the qualitative assumptions, the method, the approach, the paradigm, and the worldview that qualitative evaluation invites and demands if someone is going to be able to engage in it fully." Formal training for the committee included informational presentations at committee meetings and a first-day in-country reorientation on process and tools. Role modeling, continuous mentoring, and ongoing discussions provided opportunities for informal training. Every member of the IOM staff also received a copy of *Qualitative Research and Evaluation Methods* by Michael Quinn Patton (Patton, 2002), which Knight said proved useful for answering questions that arose during the evaluation.

The evaluation team used purposeful sampling for the selection of countries to visit and whom to interview within the countries based on a list of considerations determined by data requirements. Except when prevented by diplomatic protocol, interviews were arranged directly by the evaluation team and not by PEPFAR staff. Knight noted that the team conducted almost 400 interviews in total, including individuals with direct experience with PEPFAR in 13 countries and individuals involved in headquarters management within PEPFAR as well as in the global response to HIV. On country visits, team members received a country visit toolkit comprising a daily agenda for each team member, the interview field note format, a post-interview debriefing form, interview guides, an informed consent script, a guide to evaluation topics, and interview team roles and responsibilities. To support self-awareness through reflection and reflexivity, team members were encouraged to keep a personal journal and to discuss as a team any issues that could affect interviewing and listening skills as well as the interpretation of the data.

The overarching qualitative evaluation question was, "What is PEPFAR's contribution to the global HIV/AIDS response?" From that starting point, 10 questions emerged covering various aspects of four key evaluation areas: PEPFAR operations, implementation, effects, and transition to sustainability. Each question was formulated into smaller open-ended questions, and subsets of interview questions were selected based on the interviewee. For example, on the subject of knowledge management, the questions were designed to identify how knowledge and information were managed in order to monitor the activities and effects of the program. For the interviewer, this question led to an open-ended request for interviewees to describe the data they collect related to HIV/AIDS programs. If needed, the interviewers could use prompts such as "How do you manage the data you collect?" or "How do you use the data you collect?" Knight says these prompts were merely memory triggers and were not meant to try to direct the interviewee's response.

The accuracy of the data collection process was ensured at a number of levels. Knight explained that for in-depth qualitative interviews the PEPFAR evaluation team used end-of-interview summaries with the participants as an immediate assurance that they had been heard accurately. The team then conducted debriefings after each interview, at 1–2 day intervals, and at the end of each week in the field. Interview notes were reconciled among at least two team members, and audio recordings and transcripts were also used for some interviews. On a broader level, for the PEPFAR evaluation a database was used to log all interviews, and an audit trail tracked ongoing design decisions, data collection, and data analysis.

In closing, Knight said that the team members found that relationships within the team were valuable when challenging each other on issues relating to data acquisition or when providing critiques of ongoing data interpretation.

THE VALUE OF QUALITATIVE METHODS

Qualitative methods can reframe, explore different perspectives, and facilitate, said Anastasia Catsambas, president of EnCompass LLC. That last item—facilitate—is particularly important in the types of evaluations that she conducts, because they tend to be highly participatory. "People think participatory means just sitting around and participating, but *participatory* to us means very structured, very deliberate activities," she said. These activities have agendas, including structured discussions that get biases on the table and create interactions that lead to learning, which can be documented and incorporated into the evaluation.

Turning to the issue of reframing, Catsambas discussed the use of outcome mapping, which she and colleagues used to help the Saving Newborn Lives program reframe its understanding of its role as a catalyst or change agent. Outcome mapping, she said, starts by examining a program's activities in terms of its sphere of control—the things it controls and for which it is accountable. It then moves to the sphere of influence, which examines how the program influences changes in the behavior and actions of partners and stakeholders. Finally, this type of analysis looks at the sphere of interest, which for this program would be changes in the supply and demand for newborn care and newborn health.

Using the framework helped the Saving Newborn Lives program to think in terms of priorities and where it will get the biggest impact in terms of value added. For example, the program was criticized for conducting research, and the framework freed them to accept that research was not where its competitive advantage was high. The end result was that Saving Newborn Lives changed its emphasis from acting as a catalyst for introducing newborn health activities—which involved research, translating evidence into advocacy, launching information campaigns, trying to influence policy, and similar activities—to one that focuses on its catalytic role in scaling up newborn care. With its new emphasis, the program is focused on building newborn health into the maternal-child continuum, mobilizing communities, and promoting sharing of evidence and the spread of newborn health practices to engage a wider audience. Catsambas said that the program seized on this new approach and implemented it before the evaluation was complete.

To illustrate the role of qualitative methods in exploring perspectives, Catsambas discussed an evaluation her company, EnCompass, did of PEPFAR's activities in the eastern Caribbean region. From the start, she and her team observed that the U.S. government and the 13 countries had a different perspective on why the program was not achieving the desired effects. Both perspectives were real, she explained, and when the parties received the draft report they both contended that the other side was represented better in the evaluation. Through a process called appreciative inquiry, the two sides came to realize that they needed to stop thinking about the evaluation and instead focus on how they would work together more effectively in the future. The evaluators as facilitators need to stay appreciative, affirm all realities, be respectfully honest, and be open to different conclusions than they made originally, she explained.

Catsambas explained the idea behind appreciative inquiry. "Appreciative inquiry starts with the premise that something works, even if it's the exception," she said, "and it starts by identifying an affirmative topic of excellence that we want to inquire about." Next comes the inquiry phase, which uses facilitated dyad interviews and group interpretation of the shared data. "It is basically storytelling, but it's not static like storytelling," Catsambas said. "What you want to do is to see what does this system look like at its best dynamic?"

The inquiry phase is followed by a visioning process, a design phase, and then an innovation phase, which she characterized as the hardest step in appreciative inquiry. "The innovation phase is where you are really talking about the design components of the future, and this is where you get a lot of great ideas for indicators," said Catsambas.

The final step is implementation. The process develops culture competence, thereby contributing to implementation, because people tell stories in their own language with their own pictures. It also preserves everyone's voice, which increases both participation and buy-in while promoting a whole-systems view of the issues.

During the discussion that followed her presentation, Catsambas commented that storytelling is an important component of qualitative data gathering because it represents someone's expert experience. As an example, she said that when using appreciative inquiry methods, it is possible to solicit stories about exceptional results and get valuable details on what factors contributed to those results.

OTHER TOPICS RAISED IN DISCUSSION

The discussion session focused largely on the nitty-gritty of conducting interviews and analyzing responses. In response to a question about translation issues, Knight emphasized the importance of sharing key points with an interviewee to make sure a conversation was captured accurately. She also noted that it can be very difficult to use transcripts because of difficulties with translations. In her project, two or three people conducted interviews, with one person taking notes and the others checking those notes afterward.

Several people in the session stated they do not use audio recordings for these and other reasons. However, others remarked on the value of a recording, even if it is used just to check on notes. Some points can only be derived from repeated reading of a transcript. Also, even conscientious interviewers can get tired and lose information if they are relying solely on notes. One participant pointed to the value of tablets with which notes can be written and stored electronically, which also can facilitate analysis.

In addition, several workshop participants discussed whether it is better to bring in people from outside a country to do interviews or hire local people to do interviews. Both options have advantages and disadvantages. Local people may be less trained in qualitative research but are often much more versed in the nuances of a setting. Local people can be trained to do interviews, which builds capacity within a country, because then they are a source of interviewing expertise. At the same time, local evaluation associations are increasing in number and can be a source of trained interviewers. Also, local people may be able to do the interviews while outside researchers do the analysis.

Qualitative research can be complicated by the fact that some interviewees are more observant than others, and some interviewers are more capable of eliciting useful responses. One participant noted that this indicates why it can be so valuable to have groups of interviewers talk to groups of interviewees. Though such data gathering, similar to focus groups, raises additional issues, it gives people a chance to hear each other and augment or amend what is said.

Participants also discussed the value of open-ended questions, which can produce information unlikely to surface with more focused questions. However, the responses can be more complex and time consuming to analyze. Software for qualitative research can help with such analyses, one participant observed, even with complex responses.

7

Applying Quantitative Methods to Evaluation on a Large Scale

Important Points Made by the Speakers

- Final health outcomes often are not measured in large evaluations, but intermediate progress that is measured does not always map to health improvements.
- New methods of studying population health are becoming available, such as gathering data from disease registries, demographic surveillance sites, or household surveys.
- Though modeling can be complex, the effort can pay dividends throughout the design, implementation, and evaluation of a large-scale intervention.
- Extended cost-effectiveness analysis can look at equity issues such as distributional or financial risk protection issues.

Quantitative methods are one foundation of evaluations of large-scale, complex, multi-national initiatives. Yet many difficult decisions must be made in deciding on and implementing these methods, as pointed out by the presenters at the concurrent session on quantitative methods.

OUTCOMES MATTER

What are the possible outcomes of a large-scale evaluation? Eran Bendavid, assistant professor of medicine at Stanford University, said that they fall into three categories: operational outcomes, output outcomes, and health proxy outcomes. The health arena, he said, is fortunate to have well-circumscribed health outcomes such as all-cause and disease-specific mortality, disease prevalence or incidence, and quality-of-life measures. Often, however, these final outcomes are not measured in large evaluations, raising the question of whether such outcomes are important to the evaluation of global health initiatives. Bendavid believes the answer to that question is yes because intermediate progress may not map to health improvements. There is a great deal to be said "for surprises and unexpected results," he said. "Final outcomes are critical."

As an example of this type of surprise, he cited some unexpected findings with regard to the effects of lowering blood glucose levels in patients with type 2 diabetes. Medical dogma held that intensive therapy to lower blood glucose was unquestionably good, yet a study conducted by the Action to Control Cardiovascular Risk in Diabetes Study Group (Action to Control Cardiovascular Risk in Diabetes Study Group et al., 2008) to confirm that belief found that the use of intensive therapy to target glycated hemoglobin levels increased mortality compared to standard therapy and did not reduce cardiovascular events.

Bendavid said that measuring final outcomes should be a critical piece of an evaluation because it is necessary for comparative effectiveness and value determinations. As to why it is rare to see final outcomes reported in an evaluation, Bendavid said that based on what he has heard from participants at this workshop there are a number of reasons. One was that context matters, and that it is hard to attribute final outcomes to these heterogeneous and complex programs. Other reasons he heard included that there is not enough time or money, and that existing findings and methods are adequate and, therefore, there is no need to evaluate health outcomes.

Data for health outcomes can come from a primary data collection effort such as those conducted by the Poverty Action Lab and the Institute for Poverty Action or by national programs such as the Mexican Seguro Popular evaluation. Aggregated data from sources such as the World Bank or the World Malaria Reports can provide health outcomes data, as can existing microdata, such as demographic surveillance sites and household surveys. When available for a study country, the DHS, said Bendavid, are a great source of long-term, high-quality data, though the use of DHS data can be challenging because of timing—the surveys are administered on average every 4–5 years—and because the measurements are mostly on total child and maternal mortality and not specific diseases of interest.

But Bendavid queried whether DHS could be used to provide health outcomes data. He gave a scenario where that may be possible, using a hypothetical PEPFAR intervention using treatment as a means of preventing HIV transmission. Testing such an intervention in clinical trials that measured incidence and mortality reduction would be an enormously expensive operation, he explained, but it might be possible to use DHS instead to follow the results of the intervention. "If implementation is staggered over 1–2 years and if, during this period, you can field three to four DHS waves prior to and during the staggered implementation, and if during this time you measure all-cause adult mortality, HIV-related adult mortality, regional incidence rates, and viral suppression rates, you would have a very strong design that would piggyback on the data collection effort," said Bendavid. "Considering the cost of many of the trials that are ongoing just for looking at the potential effectiveness of treatment as prevention for HIV, this kind of an effort could be quite an attractive alternative option."

There are also new ways of studying population health that are appearing in the literature. One example is the registry based randomized trial, in which a large-scale randomized trial builds on an existing registry of observational data to identify and enroll patients without duplicating the collection of existing data (Lauer and D'Agostino, 2013). While this particular proposal is aimed at resource-rich countries, Bendavid suggested that it would be possible to expand DHS at some sites to allow testing the effects of implementing large and complex programs. Doing so would require some up-front investment, he said, but there could be substantial downstream reward given the much lower cost of collecting data in a health registry compared to the cost of recruiting participants for a clinical trial.

MATHEMATICAL MODELING AS A TOOL FOR PROGRAM EVALUATION

Charlotte Watts, head of the Social and Mathematical Epidemiology Group and founding director of the Gender, Violence, and Health Centre in the Department for Global Health and Development at the London School of Hygiene and Tropical Medicine, began her presentation with a brief discussion of how mathematical modeling can be used for an evaluation. First, she differentiated infectious disease modeling, which uses systems of equations to describe how an infectious disease might spread through a particular population, from statistical modeling intended to draw inferences from the data. These systems of mathematical equations can be used to describe the likelihood over time that different individuals might become infected with a disease. For example, HIV modeling can be used to explain how disease develops over time and how that affects the levels of antiretroviral therapy that will be needed or the mortality rates in a population. She explained that mathematical modeling is especially useful with infectious diseases such as HIV where it may not be possible to measure disease impact directly or where the available data measure trends in HIV prevalence or sexual behavior rather than the actual change in HIV incidence. Disease transmission modeling is also useful when the goal is to estimate broader, dynamic benefits of an intervention on subsequent chains of transmission among people not directly reached by the intervention (for example, behavior change that might have resulted in averted infections) and for obtaining estimates of cumulative, long-term benefits of infections averted for the purpose of cost-benefit and cost-effectiveness analyses.

Developing a useful disease transmission model for a specific setting is a multistep process. The first step in this compartmental deterministic modeling involves mapping out the different components that are interacting with one another within the context of the intervention. The components are then formulated mathematically so they can be coded to create the model. Watts noted that mathematical modelers are getting more sophisticated about incorporating measures of uncertainty associated with key inputs into their models that help capture what should be reflected into subsequent impact projections. With sampling methods that capture different combinations of potential model inputs, they then test the model using setting-specific epidemiological data (i.e., HIV prevalence) to identify which of the combinations actually fit the real HIV prevalence data that they have. This allows them to compare projections of transmission with or without the intervention to project the intervention impact and associated uncertainty.

Though the mathematics behind a model can be complex to set up, there is increased interest in applying this type of modeling as it can be useful throughout the design, implementation, and evaluation of a large-scale intervention. In the formative and early-stage planning phase, mathematical modeling can be used to predict what the impact might be when an intervention or technology is added to an existing health system to determine if the intervention is worth pursuing, how long it might take to show an effect, and whether the intervention should focus on specific populations. At this stage, explained Watts, mathematical modeling can be used to give project developers a sense of whether the size of the intervention they are planning matches the goals of the intervention in terms of the size of the desired effect. At the small-scale implementation phase of a program, mathematical modeling can take real data about an intervention's initial effectiveness to provide an idea of other settings in which this intervention could work and to explore how possible refinements to the intervention might increase its impact when the intervention moves into the large-scale delivery phase.

As an example of how mathematical modeling was used to influence early-stage thinking about program delivery and planning, Watts discussed a project that was going to introduce new microbicides as a means of reducing HIV incidence. For this project, mathematical models were used to project the effect of different introduction and uptake rates of the microbicides on the reduction of HIV incidence. This modeling effort predicted that delays in the delivery of the intervention could result in lower coverage rates and significantly reduce the intervention's potential impact on incidence. This is important information, Watts noted, that can help focus policy discussions on how to use mathematical modeling to develop targets and think through the scale of implementation needed to achieve the desired impact of an intervention.

In another example, Watts showed how mathematical modeling can be used to explore how the effects of an intervention will vary when implemented in different epidemic settings. In this case, she and her colleagues modeled the impact of microbicide on HIV transmission in Cotonou, Benin, where HIV prevalence is low and the epidemic is concentrated among vulnerable groups, compared to Hillbrow, South Africa, where HIV prevalence is much higher and the epidemic is more generalized in the population. The mathematical model projected that the same level of microbicide use would cause a much greater reduction in HIV incidence in Cotonou than in Hillbrow. However, the cumulative number of infections averted would be much greater in Hillbrow than in Cotonou, due in part to higher initial incidence in Hillbrow (Vickerman et al., 2006). Thus, mathematical modeling can provide interesting and useful information for understanding the potential impact of an intervention in different epidemiologic settings. Lastly, Watts noted that this type of modeling also can be used to create counterfactual situations to predict the course of an epidemic in the absence of a particular intervention. The counterfactual projections can then be compared to the projected outcome with the intervention implemented.

In summary, Watts said that mathematical modeling is an extremely powerful tool for exploring what-if questions and for both advocacy and rigorous evaluation. It is admittedly a complex technique with many underlying assumptions, and she noted that the modeling field is only just starting to develop guidelines for detailing those assumptions in publications so it becomes less of a "black box" activity. Mathematical modeling "is dependent on good data and strong collaborations with programs," she said, adding, "We could be using modeling far more than we are currently, both to inform the design and planning of programs, as well as for evaluation." She noted, too, that the most effective approach to bringing mathematical modeling into program activities is to involve mathematicians at the outset in a multidisciplinary evaluation team, in part to identify the data that will be needed to inform the model and be collected as part of the evaluation strategy.

EXTENDED COST-EFFECTIVENESS ANALYSIS

In the final presentation of the concurrent session, Rachel Nugent, director of the Disease Control Priorities Network at the University of Washington's Department of Global Health, discussed her team's approach to using economic modeling, together with other analytical tools such as the epidemiological and mathematical models that Watts discussed, to answer some of the what-if questions relating to economic outcomes of health interventions in the third edition of the Disease Control Priorities in Developing Countries program. The objectives of the program, which is part of the larger Disease Control Priorities Network, are to inform allocation of resources across interventions and health delivery platforms, provide a comprehensive review of the efficacy and effectiveness of priority health interventions, and advance knowledge and the practice of analytical methods for economic evaluation of health interventions. The work that Nugent discussed emerged from the third objective.

"The starting premise for this work," said Nugent, "is that health decision makers are making choices in a complex environment with limited information." Economists have something to offer health decision makers, she added, but economists need to move beyond the standard cost-effectiveness analysis. "There are many 'well-known and well-justified' criticisms of cost-effective analysis," she said, "but one of them is simply that it doesn't provide sufficient information of the type that health ministries and other decision makers need. It's often too narrow about a given intervention." To address this shortcoming, she and her colleagues are trying to find a middle ground between cost-effectiveness analysis and cost-benefit analysis to develop what she called a dashboard of economic outcome measures that can be compared across a broad range of intervention choices. These economic outcome measures revolve around adding to the evidence base for equity and financial risk protection for the users of services.

Nugent noted that previous incarnations of the Disease Control Priorities in Developing Countries program were instrumental in advancing understanding of the economic aspects of health and what economic information is useful to inform health decisions. The World Health Report 2000 (WHO, 2000) was also a seminal document, in part because it not only exposed how poorly the U.S. health system was doing on a comparative basis, but also because it asserted that health systems are supposed to provide more than just health. "Yes, health systems should provide improved health outcomes, but they should also provide economic outcomes," said Nugent. Such economic outcomes include prevention of medical impoverishment and fairness in the final contribution toward health. Along those lines, she and her colleagues are hoping that the measures they are developing can help inform the discussion about universal health care and how to design a basic insurance package taking into account the needs of individual countries.

One aspect of Nugent's work has been to move from cost-effectiveness analysis to extended cost-effectiveness analysis that looks at equity issues, such as the distributional consequences across wealth strata of populations and the financial risk protection benefits for households (Verguet et al., 2014). As an example of the use of extended cost-effectiveness analysis, Nugent discussed its application to an analysis of a human papilloma virus (HPV) vaccination policy in China. She observed that "You have to look at the vaccination and then cervical cancer screening and treatment all together, because if you just look at one of them you're going to miss a lot of the important impacts. They have to go together to really be able to talk about what you get out of a policy of HPV vaccination." The starting point for this analysis is the introduction of the technology and the policy of a government subsidy for HPV vaccination and a set of expected impacts, measured by the number of cancer deaths averted; household expenditures, measured by cancer treatment expenditures that are averted; and financial risk protection benefits, measured by the relative importance of treatment expenditures to the household budget. These effects were measured by income quintile, but Nugent explained that they could have been measured by urban versus rural status or male versus female to see if the policy favors one sex over the other. "There are different ways we could disaggregate the population if we have the data to measure different distributional aspects," she said. This example's analysis showed that China's policy will favor poorer families in terms of the savings to lower income people as a much higher percentage of their income.

OTHER TOPICS RAISED IN DISCUSSION

During the discussion period, Bendavid was asked about the use of demographic surveillance sites (DSSs) for interventions research. He explained that these are relatively small or constrained communities that can provide very high-quality data. But it can be hard to draw general conclusions from such specific settings, even though in some cases data from these sites have been used to great effect. Increasing the number of sites in a country could increase the value of this information, he added.

Watts expanded on the use of counterfactual parameters, which are essential for modeling the impact of an intervention. The process of choosing what data goes into a model is becoming much more sophisticated and transparent, she said, but it is also complicated by the multiplicity of programs and program elements. Models inevitably must trade complexity for simplicity. By clearly articulating these trade-offs in published documents, they can be open to questioning and review.

Nugent emphasized the importance of thinking broadly about value questions in health resource allocations. Value for money can mean different things to different people. Overall efficiency is one measure, but so are the effect on households and distributional effects.

8

Analysis Through Triangulation and Synthesis to Interpret Data in a Mixed Methods Evaluation

```
┌─────────────────────────────────────────────────────────┐
│              Important Points Made by the Speakers        │
│                                                           │
│  •  Synthesis and triangulation among multiple sources of infor- │
│     mation and multiple types of methods can strengthen the qual- │
│     ity and credibility of the evidentiary support for findings and │
│     recommendations, especially in complex interventions where │
│     any single data source will have inherent limitations.         │
│  •  A theory of change provides an analytical framework for tri- │
│     angulation, but the theory may need to change as data are │
│     analyzed.                                              │
│  •  Triangulation has benefited from the development of protocols, │
│     procedures, and methodologies.                        │
│  •  Triangulation benefits from multidisciplinary teams of │
│     investigators.                                        │
└─────────────────────────────────────────────────────────┘
```

In this session, the workshop explored some of the key considerations of data analysis and interpretation for a complex, mixed methods evaluation, and particularly the use of triangulation and synthesis among multiple complementary sources of information and multiple evaluators to enhance the robustness, quality, and credibility of the evidence for evaluation conclusions and recommendations.

Triangulation, explained session moderator Carlo Carugi, who is senior evaluation officer and team leader at the Global Environmental Facility

(GEF), refers to the use of multiple sources of qualitative information, quantitative information, and data collection and analysis methods to arrive at evaluation findings or conclusions. "In research, [triangulation] is usually done either to validate the results in a study or to deepen and widen one's understanding and insights into study results." He noted that the literature contains several articles describing how data, theories, and methods are triangulated in a range of fields, but there are also articles critical of triangulation because of its lack of theoretic or empirical justification and its ad hoc nature. The development of standardized protocols, procedures, and methodologies for triangulation have helped address this criticism.

TRIANGULATION IN THE GLOBAL ENVIRONMENTAL FACILITY

Carugi described the use of triangulation in the GEF, which is a partnership among 183 countries with international institutions, civil society organizations, and the private sector to address global environmental issues while supporting national sustainable development initiatives. In the evaluation process, methodological triangulation is most commonly used in situations where data are unreliable or scarce. For example, the GEF uses triangulation among methods and observers in its country portfolio evaluations. Triangulation reduces the risk of giving excessive importance to the results of one method over those of the other methods used to analyze the collected data.

Common challenges the GEF faces when evaluating country portfolios, Carugi said, include the absence of country program objectives and indicators over the 20 or so years of a typical evaluation and the scarcity or unreliability of national statistics on environmental indicators and data series over that time frame, particularly in the least developed countries. He noted, too, that because the GEF is a partnership institution, it has no control authority over the national monitoring and evaluation systems that feed data into the GEF's central monitoring information system hub. There are also challenges in evaluating the effects of GEF projects and establishing attribution, as well as the intrinsic difficulties in defining the GEF portfolio of projects prior to undertaking an evaluation.

To address these challenges, the GEF has adopted an iterative and inclusive approach that engages stakeholders during the evaluation process to help identify and address information and data gaps. This step is essential at the country level, said Carugi. The GEF conducts original evaluative research, including theory-based approaches, during the evaluation to assess progress toward desired impacts in the face of sparse data. It also uses qualitative methods and mixes emerging evidence with available quantitative data through systematic triangulation with the ultimate goal of identifying evaluation findings.

Carugi said the GEF's country portfolio evaluations are all conducted in a standardized way using standard terms of reference and questions for comparability purposes. The initial terms of reference are made country specific through stakeholder consultation during a scoping mission to the country. The GEF then uses a standard set of data gathering methods and tools that include methods such as desk and literature reviews, portfolio analyses, and interviews, in addition to GEF-specific methods, such as analyses of a country's environmental legal framework and reviews of outcomes to impact, which is a theory-based approach to examine the progress from outcomes to impact. All of these methods are deployed within the context of an evaluation matrix that the GEF develops for each evaluation.

The evaluation matrix then feeds into a triangulation matrix. "We categorize the evaluative evidence in three major research areas of perceptions, validation, and documentation," said Carugi, explaining that perceptions, while not always reflecting reality, need to be accounted for in these evaluations (see Figure 8-1). In the triangulation process, the evaluation team

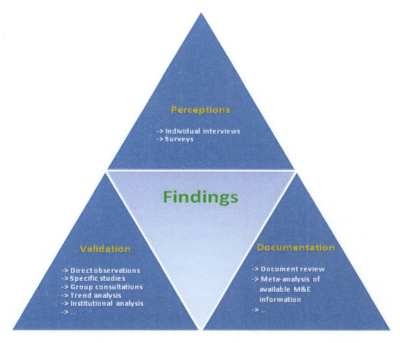

FIGURE 8-1 Three major areas of evaluative evidence in the Global Environmental Facility country program evaluations, as presented by Carugi.
NOTE: M&E = monitoring and evaluation.
SOURCE: Carugi, 2014.

brainstorms question by question to populate the matrix and discuss which findings are real and which need further analysis. "After the triangulation brainstorming meeting, we go back to the drawing board and try to confirm or challenge the key preliminary evaluation findings and try to identify what we can do to fill in the missing key preliminary evaluation findings," said Carugi.

DEVELOPING A DEEPER AND WIDER UNDERSTANDING OF RESULTS

As described previously, the AMFm evaluation, said Catherine Goodman, senior lecturer in health economics and policy in the Department of Global Health and Development at the London School of Hygiene and Tropical Medicine, was a before-and-after study that did not have control areas. The study used outlet surveys at baseline and endline, household survey data for some of the countries being evaluated, and documentation of key contextual factors. The focus of Goodman's talk was on using triangulation of the data gathered through different sources to deepen and widen the AMFm evaluation team's understanding of the evaluation results.

The AMFm evaluation team developed a theory of change to depict the causal pathways through which AMFm interventions were intended to work. This theory of change was used to target the collection of quantitative and qualitative data that would be used to prepare case studies for each country. To understand the AMFm implementation processes and contextual factors within each country, the evaluation team collected qualitative data through key stakeholder interviews with public- and private-sector actors and reviewed key documents. The evaluation team also used some quantitative data from the outlet surveys on process-related outcomes such as coverage of training and exposure to communications messages. The evaluators analyzed these data separately for each country case study and then synthesized findings across countries.

The country case studies allowed the evaluation team to understand the level of AMFm implementation within each country and to compare implementation strength across countries and these data were helpful for interpreting the survey results related to outcomes and key success metrics. For example, Madagascar only met one success metric out of six, but the data from the case study revealed some process and contextual reasons for the country's relatively poor performance. Orders for medication were low to begin with because of low confidence among importers, and the information and communications campaign was limited because in-country regulators decided that direct-to-consumer advertising was inappropriate and banned the practice 1 month into the program. In addition, several activities in the country muddled the baseline measures, and a coup d'état and deterioration of the country's economy during the pilot study further complicated matters. "I am not sure if I could say which one of these is the most important or if you were to remove one of those problems things would have been okay. It is not possible to really go that far, but it does help us identify some of the factors contributing to the poor performance."

While triangulating data from multiple sources deepened the evaluators' understanding of evaluation results within countries, synthesizing the findings across countries contributed to an understanding of how an AMFm intervention could work in other countries in the future by identifying the key factors that contributed to strong performance as well as those associated with weaker performance. She noted that one of the lessons learned from this type of evaluation is how important it is to document the process of implementation through a theory of change model when such a large-scale, complex intervention is being implemented in a messy, real-world setting. "Context was incredibly important," she said, and "context probably made the most crucial difference between countries" in terms of performance.

TRIANGULATION IN PRACTICE

One of the major challenges inherent in multidisciplinary science, said Jonathan Simon, Robert A. Knox Professor and director of the Center for Global Health and Development at Boston University, is working with the multidisciplinary team of investigators needed to do good multidisciplinary science. One ingredient of success, he continued, is respectful skepticism. The President's Malaria Initiative evaluation team took an approach in which for every key issue it matched the team member who had the dominant relevant expertise with somebody who had completely different expertise, or as Simon put it, "somebody who would just take a different perspective such that when our team got together there were two presentations of their interpretation." This led to a richer understanding of the analysis, which Simon described as "a healthy approach."

Simon briefly discussed why discordant results do not worry him. Timing, for example, is one factor that can produce discordance if events such as management changes occur during the course of an evaluation. "On all of these evaluations, we are looking at 3-, 5-, and 8-year periods, and we should be very careful about the timing of the slice of information from the informant or from the survey, given that these are retrospective looks." He suggested performing an analysis of discordance that looks at the different sources of information, the different methods being used, and the different levels of analysis to try to make sure that findings are as rich as possible.

APPROACHES TO TRIANGULATION

Sangeeta Mookherji, assistant professor in the Department of Global Health at George Washington University, spoke about the lessons she has learned conducting large-scale mixed methods evaluations. She began by saying one of the biggest concerns with this type of evaluation is ensuring that data quality is as good as it can be in order to have the highest confidence possible in the results of the evaluation. "We need to think about validity and reliability regardless of what method we are using, but triangulation is one method to help with these things," said Mookherji. She added that there are different ways of doing triangulation and that "you need to be mindful of choosing an appropriate way depending on what your objective is." The theory of change is the analytical framework for triangulation or any other analytical method used, said Mookherji. However, she noted, "You have to be willing to also approach your theory with healthy skepticism and make the modifications and changes as you learn from your data and learn through your analysis and validation."

Drawing from her experiences conducting multiple mixed methods evaluations, she noted that triangulation approaches, or processes for integrating or combining qualitative and quantitative data, can vary depending on the questions being addressed by the evaluation. It can also depend on the data sources and the formats of the data, including the available software and other tools for working with the data.

For a multicountry case study of routine immunization in sub-Saharan Africa funded by the Bill & Melinda Gates Foundation, which was asking what has driven improvements in immunization performance, Mookherji described how the evaluation team created systematic formats that every analyst used to extract information from the raw data and put it into categories that they then grouped by theme. "That is how we started to [ask] are we actually reaching consensus on an understanding of a key preliminary finding? [The findings then] went back to the external evaluation advisory group, as well as the larger team and the country teams, for validation," Mookherji explained. This integration process, she said, enabled the team to understand what it was validating and how it was using triangulation.

Mookherji then spoke about synthesizing knowledge across countries. "Are there generalizable and relevant findings that you can draw out of the context and use in a wider perspective? That is really where I find that we need to do better with mixed methodologies," she said. "We need to articulate what we need to do to ensure legitimate synthesis and legitimate drawing of more generalizable findings." Validating preliminary findings within the evaluation team is an important first step, she said, and for that it is important to have divergent perspectives within the team to continually challenge any conclusions being made. Mookherji added that she has teams doing qualitative interviews so that two people are listening to every response and can make sure they both heard the same thing. She also includes an articulated process for alternative theory testing to ensure her team challenges its assumptions about the pathways by which an outcome or impact was achieved or not achieved. Finally, looking at the findings in terms of context is important when synthesizing findings.

LESSONS FROM THE IOM'S PEPFAR EVALUATION

In this session's final presentation, Bridget Kelly, senior program officer with the IOM Board on Global Health and the IOM/NRC Board on Children, Youth, and Families, spoke about the many layers of embedded and integrated triangulation in the IOM's evaluation of PEPFAR, for which she was the study co-director. The many layers were needed to deal with different data sources, different investigators, and different subsets of the initiative. She noted that this analysis sometimes came up with discordant results that were not discarded but instead reported along with any evidentiary support for such findings. However, the overall process sought to find resonances among data sources to enhance trust in the reliability, credibility, and applicability of conclusions (see Figure 8-2).

One issue with the analysis, she noted, was that few data sources were available consistently across the entire PEPFAR program. The evaluation team did not try to integrate data. Instead, said Kelly, "We thought about integration happening at the level of analyses and interpretation," acknowledging that "there is sometimes a gray area between what is data and what is analysis because you are thinking about what the data mean even as you are looking at the data."

Instead of integrating data, the evaluation team focused on using rigorous methods for data collection and analysis within each type of data and matching the appropriate analytical methods to the different types of data. It was important, she explained, to document clearly what analytical methods were used for each type of data to ensure that the analysis was as purposeful and rigorous as possible. You want to have "mixed methods, and not just mixed up methods," said Kelly, borrowing a phrase used previously by Larry Aber of New York University.

One strength of the evaluation process was that with a single institution managing the entire evaluation, the staff were working closely together at all times, which enabled the team to engage in frequent group discussions. The team also engaged in an iterative process of reading and responding to questions from committee members and each other that enabled the development of narratives that were consistent within countries and from which broader findings could be drawn. Kelly noted that this type of triangulation

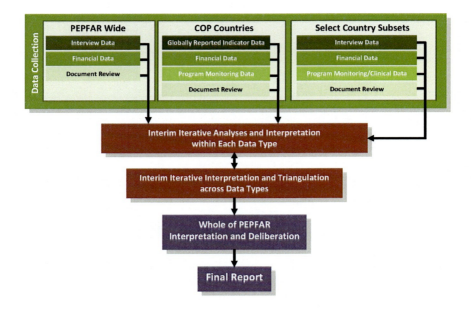

FIGURE 8-2 The PEPFAR evaluation used multiple types and sources of data in an iterative triangulation process for integrated analysis and interpretation.
Note: COP = Country Operational Plan.
SOURCE: IOM, 2013.

across evaluators within the entire team of committee members, consultants, and staff continued throughout the entire analysis and deliberation phase of the evaluation.

Because this process was highly iterative, in some cases it resulted in having to go back to the original data or asking for more data. For example, once the team examined all of the program monitoring data that were available across the countries that were within the scope of the evaluation, it was able to get a sense of how limited the findings would be from that data source alone. As a result, the team requested data from other sources, such as CDC. From the team's perspective, this triangulation process strengthened the quality and credibility of the evidentiary support for its findings and recommendations.

One drawback to this approach is that it is time consuming, said Kelly. At any one time, the evaluation team had 8 staff, 3 consultants, and 20 committee members. "That is a lot of people thinking, and ultimately all 20 of our committee members had to reach consensus on our conclusions and recommendations," she noted. Not only was this process time consuming, but it was also operationally challenging because it forced the IOM staff to plan for draft data presentations that the committee could examine and respond to in a way that was both iterative and efficient.

OTHER TOPICS RAISED IN DISCUSSION

During the discussion session, several workshop participants raised the question of whether triangulation is possible between just two sources of data, such as one source of quantitative and one source of qualitative data. Several panelists agreed that two sources is often not enough to have confidence in results. "That is why I think multiple members of our panel said it is multiple methods, not always mixed methods," said Simon. Kelly noted, however, that it depends on the data available and the evaluation question. Sometimes it might take eight data sources to trust a conclusion, while on narrow issues one reliable data source may be sufficient.

Mookherji emphasized the importance of context, which sometimes gets removed in the course of analysis. At that point it becomes necessary to look at theory again and understand the effects of context. Common elements across different contexts can serve as a form of triangulation, she said, even though each setting also can have discordant elements.

In response to a question, Kelly described the process in general of arriving at consensus on the IOM committees. Recommendations are often the areas where the strongest resonance emerges among committee members, as well as areas that are most important for the study. Reports also contain information that is not necessarily at this level, though all committee members have to agree to author the final report. In some areas, it may be possible only to state findings and not progress to conclusions or recommendations.

Panelists also discussed the need for rigor when using mixed methods. Data gathering and analyses need to be as transparent as possible, said Mookherji, even if they are never completely reproducible. Publishing a protocol in advance and sticking to it is one way to achieve rigor, Goodman noted, but in an evaluation the protocol may need to change if the pathway to impacts is unclear. Data gathering and analysis may need to be iterative, though this process also can be documented. Simon observed that the level of rigor required for decision making and program improvement is not a fixed entity. Evaluators do the most rigorous analysis necessary to meet the needs of a program, and that level is highly variable. "Often we allow rigor to get in the way of utility and usefulness," he said.

9

Evolving Methods in Evaluation Science

Important Points Made by the Speakers

- Realist methods are one way to understand the mechanisms that generate outcomes and the relationship between the outcomes and the context.
- Innovative methods can make it possible to gather evaluation data in situations that would not have been amenable to analysis in the past.
- Nonexperimental, observational, and mixed methods can provide valuable evaluation information.

Many technologies, techniques, and approaches are available in evaluation science. The presenters at this concurrent sessions examined some of these evaluation approaches, including long-standing principles of evaluation science that have continuously evolved as well as new approaches that have been introduced. The speakers focused on potential application in the evaluation of complex initiatives and interventions in complex systems.

USE OF REALIST METHODS TO EVALUATE COMPLEX INTERVENTIONS AND SYSTEMS

There are two types of realist methods, said Geoff Wong, senior lecturer in primary care at Queen Mary, University of London. The first, called realist evaluation, is theory-driven evaluation in which the evaluator generates data and conducts primary research. The other, realist synthesis, which Wong said is derived from realist evaluation, is a form of systematic literature review that can be considered secondary research. In realist synthesis, the goal is more about explaining and understanding how and why an intervention works rather than looking at whether it does or does not work (Pawson, 2013).

Most large interventions have multiple interacting components that tend not to act in a linear fashion. "You can put a vast amount of effort in at one end and not necessarily get back your return" on the final desired outcome or the proximal outcomes, said Wong. Interventions are also highly dependent on the context in which they take place and on the variability associated with the fact that every intervention relies on people, from those who are the targets of the intervention to those who are on the ground delivering the intervention. As an example, he cited his experience with large smoking cessation programs, which deal with a wide range of smokers who have a variety of motivations to stop smoking, strategies for kicking the habit, and responses both to particular interventions and to when they fail any one attempt to quit smoking. In addition, those delivering the intervention have different personal approaches, further complicating the context of the intervention.

In their potential to address this complexity, realist methods differ from other methods, Wong said, by starting with an ontology based on critical realism that attempts to identify, understand, and explain causation through generative mechanisms. The idea, he said, is that interventions themselves do not necessarily cause any outcomes. Instead, what causes the outcomes are what he called mechanisms. "Mechanisms are a causal process, a driving force." For example, letting go of an object does not make it fall—gravity does. Letting go of the object is the intervention, but gravity is the mechanism. One key concept is that mechanisms can be hidden yet they are real and can be used even though they cannot be seen or touched. "None of us have ever seen gravity, but we are able to see the effects of gravity," he said. They are also context dependent—an object dropped on the moon would fall at a different velocity than an object dropped on earth.

Wong noted that these concepts enable the ability to develop a logic of analysis that depends on the mechanism. Middle-range theories that are close enough to the data to be testable can then explain the relationships between outcome, context, and mechanism.

Epistemology is another way in which realist methods differ from other methods. "How do we know something is knowledge?" Wong asked. Knowledge should be judged by assessing the processes and assumptions by which it is produced, he said. He analogized this to detective work that starts with outcomes and works backward to understand the cause. "Theories are right because they are, for example, coherent, plausible, and repeatedly successful." From the ontological perspective of a realist, the world is stratified. There are layers that give the world depth, with mechanisms operating at a layer that may not be immediately observable. As a result, Wong said, controlling for context may be neither possible nor desirable because doing so "may in fact be stripping out the thing that is an important trigger to the mechanism."

Wong finished his remarks by noting that it helps to have some grounding in the philosophy of science to understand the basis of realist methods and how best to apply them. The realist synthesis has quality reporting standards and training materials available on the web, and there is a discussion group for anyone interested in realist research, he said.[1]

INNOVATIVE DESIGNS FOR COMPLEX QUESTIONS

Emmanuela Gakidou, professor of global health and director of education and training at the Institute for Health Metrics and Evaluation at the University of Washington, discussed three complex interventions that she and her colleagues are evaluating using innovative designs. The first project, Salud Mesoamerica 2015, is a 5-year, public–private partnership with multiple funders whose purpose is to improve health indicators for the poorest quintile of people living in Mesoamerica—Mexico from Chiapas plus all of Central America—using results-based financing as a way to implement the intervention. The objectives of the evaluation, Gakidou explained, are to assess if countries are reaching the initiative's targets as agreed to between each country and the Inter-American Development Bank, the project's managing organization, and to evaluate the impact of the specific components of all interventions in each country.

The evaluation design includes a baseline measurement prior to the intervention and three follow-up measurements over the course of the 5-year project, with intervention and control groups in most countries. To deal with the complexity of the project, Gakidou and her colleagues are using what they consider to be innovative ways of conducting measurements, including sampling populations at high risk so they can have enough of a sample size to make inferences at the end, capturing data electronically, evaluating the quality of the data during data entry, and evaluating project implementation. Another innovation, she noted, is linking the health facilities where households are receiving care with the information from household surveys to provide a flow of information between the supply side and the demand side for these communities. "We also do a lot of health facility observations and medical record review information extraction from charts,

---

[1] More information is available at http://www.ramsesproject.org (accessed April 8, 2014).

so we don't just rely on qualitative assessments in the facilities," she said. For example, the evaluation is using dried blood spot analysis to measure immunity status in the children rather than just relying on immunization status reports from the facilities.

Next, Gakidou described the Global Alliance for Vaccines and Immunization (GAVI) full-country evaluation. The goal of this evaluation is to understand and quantify the barriers to and the drivers of immunization program improvement, including GAVI's contribution, in five countries: Bangladesh, India, Mozambique, Uganda, and Zambia. It is a 4-year prospective evaluation that started in 2013 with a $16 million budget, and it is using monitoring indicators to comprehensively evaluate inputs, process, outcomes, and impacts as well as contextual factors and equity (see Figure 9-1). Given that GAVI is not the only agency working on immunization in these five countries, the evaluation will attempt to look at the whole immunization system and GAVI's role in that system. The evaluation is also designed to answer several more specific questions about GAVI's contribution to immunization rates and, ultimately, to reductions in child mortality.

The GAVI evaluation uses a mixed methods approach to analyze quantitative and qualitative data from sources, including process evaluation, resource tracking, facility surveys, household surveys, verbal autopsies,

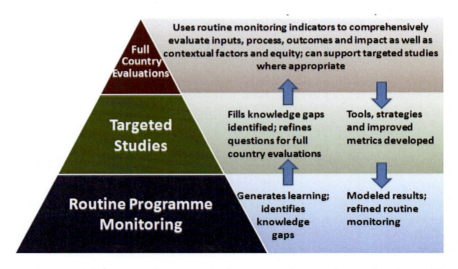

FIGURE 9-1 The GAVI Full Country Evaluation sought to understand and quantify the barriers to and drivers of immunization program improvement through routine program monitoring, targeted studies, and full country evaluations, as presented by Gakidou.
SOURCE: Printed by courtesy of the GAVI Alliance, 2010.

vaccine effectiveness assessments, small area analyses, and impact analyses. The evaluation is using existing data and, as Gakidou explained, "we're supplementing that with what we call smart primary data collection, where we piggyback on existing programs like the DHS and oversample some populations or add additional questionnaires for subsampling some populations." She observed that this saved costs for the evaluation while taking advantage of other ongoing, large-scale activities.

Finally, Gakidou discussed the evaluation of the Malaria Control Policy Assessment, funded by the Bill & Melinda Gates Foundation, which is designed to determine how much of the reduction in child mortality seen in Zambia over the past two decades is a result of scaled-up malaria control interventions. She explained that in addition to malaria control efforts—distribution of insecticide-treated bed nets and indoor residual spraying—there has been an expansion of efforts to prevent mother-to-child transmission of HIV through PEPFAR, a transformation and scale-up of immunization programs combined with the development of a new pentavalent vaccine, the introduction of child health weeks, and other health interventions new to Zambia since the mid-1990s. Contextual factors also have been at work, including economic growth and huge improvements in the education of women of reproductive age. "What we're trying to figure out is if the rate of decrease in child mortality accelerated as a result of malaria control interventions, and if so, by how much," said Gakidou.

The first step in the evaluation has been to estimate trends at the district level for all quantities of interest between 1990 and 2010. Next the evaluation will conduct causal attribution analyses looking at a number of variables addressing the entire range of health interventions and a composite measure for sociodemographic factors. Gakidou noted that there are variables that she would liked to have added to this analysis, including both malaria control and other health-related interventions that are critically linked to child mortality, but that the data are not available. Noting "We're a fairly quantitative institute where I work," she said that her team tested dozens of models, ranging from linear models to structural equation modeling, along with many combinations of interventions using random effects, fixed effects, and other approaches.

Currently, she and her colleagues are favoring a linear model with bootstrapping that includes distribution of insecticide-treated bed nets and indoor residual spraying, seven other key health interventions, and a composite measure of non-health factors. Analyzing the data using this model shows that none of the interventions stands out as being significant on its own. "You can imagine with so many things going on, it's really difficult to figure out what actually is leading to the reduction of under-5 mortality," Gakidou said. "In some ways it's not fair for somebody to ask me what has been the contribution of the malaria control scale-up to child mortality, and in some ways it's my responsibility as a quantitative analyst to say that, given this graph, I really can't tell you." A counterfactual analysis suggested that if none of these interventions had been instituted, under-five child mortality in Zambia would have been 13 percent higher in 2010, which Gakidou characterized as "a remarkable reduction and acceleration in the pace of child mortality reduction."

In closing, Gakidou said that one implication of the studies she discussed is that for broad, complex global health evaluations, retrospective evaluations are always limited by available data. "You can't go in and design your own study to answer the question, and what this means is that sometimes you can't actually answer the question you set out to answer, but you still learn a lot of valuable information along the way," she remarked. "So, as an evaluator, my pitch is that large global health programs and initiatives need to build in evaluation from the beginning, like the study on Mesoamerica that I was referring to, because the evidence base on what works and what does not work urgently needs to be expanded in our field."

COMPARATIVE SYSTEMS ANALYSIS: METHODOLOGICAL CHALLENGES AND LESSONS FROM EDUCATION RESEARCH

Education research over the past 20 years in developing countries has often been criticized by donors for being fragmented, small scale, non-cumulative, and methodologically flawed, as well as for being politically motivated, researcher driven, and of limited relevance for policy and practice, said Caine Rolleston, lecturer in education and international development at the Institute of Education, University of London. This criticism, he explained, has led to an increasing emphasis on what is considered to be the "gold standard" of experimental methods—the randomized controlled trial—but there is also a need for better evaluation of education systems through nonexperimental, observational, and mixed methods.

As an example, he discussed the Young Lives survey, a longitudinal study of 12,000 children born in two cohorts in Ethiopia, India, Peru, and Vietnam that was designed originally to look at childhood poverty.[2] In 2010, when the younger cohort of children reached age 10, Rolleston and his colleagues started including school surveys focused on math and literacy and measuring progress in learning over time. They also looked at school and teacher effectiveness using a longitudinal, within-school design, and included both the indexed children and class peers to get a balanced sample of children at the school and class level.

Rolleston noted that despite a large number of studies of the effects of observable school inputs, there is little consistent evidence of what works

---

[2] More information is available at http://www.younglives.org.uk (accessed April 8, 2014).

in terms of individual school inputs. "Not only that, but those effects that are consistently significant are pretty much the most obvious ones and don't offer a huge amount of guidance for additional programs and projects," he said. "That's partly because of the large differences in context, but also because of the very large number of variables that are included in school effectiveness studies." Nonetheless, despite the poor consistency of these findings, there are large differences in the effectiveness of education systems. "It seems that those are bound up with different kinds of system characteristics, political economy characteristics, and bundles of inputs that vary in inconsistent ways across countries," Rolleston said.

When looking at student performance data in the four countries studied in the Young Lives survey, there are clear differences in learning levels between the four systems. Children in India, for example, do not make as much progress in math as do children in Vietnam between ages 7 and 14. While there are inconsistent patterns of explanatory variables, two factors stood out: all teachers in Vietnam received formal teacher training, while 16.5 percent of teachers in India did not, and nearly a third of students in India reported that their teacher was often absent, while teacher absenteeism in Vietnam was exceedingly rare. "But assessing school quality in comparative terms between two systems is quite complex, because what you really need is to be able to measure the value added over time," said Rolleston, "To do that you need to be able to separate the effects of pupils' backgrounds from their prior attainment, which requires a longitudinal design, repeated measures of test scores at the school level, and linked data between teachers, schools, and pupil backgrounds." While difficult to achieve, Rolleston and his team successfully used these sophisticated designs for value-added analysis where they have found big differences in cross-sectional effects compared to longitudinal effects.

Another challenge in developing countries is to develop context-appropriate measures for educational performance. Rolleston and his colleagues used a package of assessments, including teacher tests and a progressive linked pupil achievement test in core subjects to provide relevant and robust measures of learning over time, including skills such as school engagement and self-confidence. They then scaled the results using latent trait models to look at change over time in a comparable way. Performing value-added analysis test results, he noted, requires an understanding of both school and teacher quality as well as methodological rigor in constructing the assessments. "This is not only a technical issue, but one very much about the relevance of the tests," Rolleston stated, adding that the design of these relevant learning metrics in developing countries "has been extremely demanding." In Ethiopia, for example, not only is the literacy level low, but there are eight linguistic groups and languages of instruction.

It also is necessary to balance national curricula and expectations with international norms in literacy and numeracy.

When the analysis of the four countries was complete, Rolleston and his colleagues were able to answer the question posed by the donor, which was what is it about Vietnam's educational system that enables it to be more effective over time? "The general lesson is that it's an equity-oriented, centralized public school system," said Rolleston. There is greater equity in the public school system, which is linked to higher performance for the majority of pupils. To achieve equity, Vietnam has an emphasis on fundamental or minimum school quality and that, he added, "means that the least advantaged pupils and the most disadvantaged areas do not suffer from as extreme a disadvantage as they do in the other countries in our study." Other important factors for Vietnam's higher levels of student performance are a greater degree of standardization in terms of curricula and textbooks that are more closely matched to pupils' learning levels and abilities, a commitment to mastery by all pupils, and the use of regular assessments.

In closing, Rolleston said that, in education, data on learning metrics in developing countries are still inadequate, that there are few rigorous assessments of students' learning performance, and that a robust longitudinal study design is needed to assess school quality. Context is also critically important to the development of a theory of change, he added.

OTHER TOPICS RAISED IN DISCUSSION

During the discussion period, the presenters turned to the issue of whether sophisticated statistics are needed to identify the effect of an intervention in a complex setting. Gakidou answered that choices made in the design and data collection can reduce the need for statistical analyses of that kind. However, the links between an intervention and outcomes need to be clearly drawn to understand causal mechanisms.

Wong pointed out that interventions are heterogeneous, not just people and settings. They should actually be seen more as a family of interventions. In that case, evaluations seek to understand why these heterogeneous inputs should produce a certain set of outcomes. The causal mechanisms, which are more universal, become the areas of focus.

Rolleston expressed interest in the application of realist evaluation to educational interventions, despite the complexities of doing so. For example, such an approach could produce insights on causal mechanisms in education that go beyond statistical associations. "Any teacher can explain to you why a particular textbook is better or worse than another. You don't need a statistical analysis for that." Wong agreed, pointing out that realist methods can help explain patterns observed in data.

10

Lessons from Large-Scale Program Evaluation on a Not-Quite-as-Large Scale

---

Important Points Made by the Speakers

- Other concurrent programs in target regions can complicate the attribution of effects to a smaller-scale intervention.
- All phases of an intervention can be treated as learning opportunities for evaluators.
- Evaluation of smaller-scale interventions during their rollout can provide valuable cause-and-effect data.
- New technologies can boost data quality and control and enable automated data harvesting and analysis.

Many of the lessons learned from evaluations of large-scale, complex multi-national initiatives can be applied as well to evaluations of smaller scale or less complex interventions. In one of the four concurrent sessions, presenters examined several of these interventions in areas of overlap with issues discussed during the rest of the workshop.

SAVING MOTHERS, GIVING LIFE STRATEGIC IMPLEMENTATION EVALUATION

The Saving Mothers, Giving Life program is a global, public–private partnership in which a consortium of six institutions, including the U.S. government, is working to reduce maternal mortality by 50 percent in four districts each in Uganda and Zambia. These two countries were chosen for phase one of this program, explained Margaret Kruk, assistant professor in health policy and management at Columbia University's Mailman School of Public Health, because they were already committed to maternal mortality reduction, had existing strategies to reduce maternal mortality, and were supportive of accelerating their programs. She noted that, after she and her team of five researchers and four faculty were commissioned as an independent evaluator of the implementation phase of the program, it took them "2 to 3 months of intense work and many trips to the countries just to describe this highly complex program." The goal of this evaluation, she added, was to inform the scale-up of this program.

One unusual aspect of this program was that it relied on CDC and USAID contractors who were already in country and who had worked in the PEPFAR program, which meant that the infrastructure already existed for getting the program up and running. "Almost overnight, they were able to turn around their existing programs to deliver these new services or support delivery of these services that were being delivered through government health clinics," said Kruk.

The evaluation examined 28 discrete activities conducted by the program in four broad areas: (1) increasing demand for services, (2) improving access to services, (3) improving the quality of services, and (4) strengthening the overall health care delivery system in the target districts. Kruk noted that one confounding factor was that other programs were ongoing in the target districts that were involved in improving access to and delivery of health services, whether it was maternal health, HIV, or child health. "It's an incredibly crowded environment in which to work both from a logistics point of view and from an attribution point of view," said Kruk. "If there is change, what part of it comes from our program versus the many, many other things that are going on?"

The aims of the evaluation, said Kruk, were to assess the extent and fidelity of the implementation of the Saving Mothers, Giving Life interventions, to assess how the partnership was functioning as a global coalition, and to identify best practices and barriers to success to improve the effectiveness of the scale-up. For an evaluation framework, the team took a traditional implementation evaluation framework and added elements to capture systems dynamics. "It was very clear that something this large is going to have ripple effects, and there are going to be nonlinearities and all sorts of complex effects," said Kruk. The evaluation took 1 year to complete and cost $1.6 million.

The issue of attribution was of particular interest to the evaluation team. "This is a massive program, so how dramatically does it change the trajectory of change that is already going on in Africa?" asked Kruk. "We know mortality is declining already. How much is this program shifting that curve even more?" To answer this question, the evaluation compared what the program achieved with what was happening in other districts. However, comparison districts were not included in the original evaluation design, so the team conducted post-test exit surveys with women who delivered in health facilities along with satisfaction surveys and obstetric knowledge tests to providers in both program and noncontiguous comparison districts. The evaluation was not funded to conduct a population survey, so the evaluation team conducted 80 focus group discussions with women to help identify any remaining barriers that inhibited or prevented women from using the program's services.

Kruk commented briefly on several aspects of the quantitative analysis phase of the evaluation, pointing out, for example, that there were challenges with measuring fidelity and quality. When all was said and done, the evaluation found that Saving Mothers, Giving Life increased provider knowledge by about 10 percent in both Uganda and Zambia after a substantial amount of training and expense. "That was a lot of investment for a 10 percent knowledge gain," said Kruk. Provider confidence, the providers' rating of quality, and the women's rating of quality showed marked increases in Uganda but little or no change in Zambia, though the program did increase women's satisfaction in Zambia but not Uganda.

Why did the program work better in Uganda despite similar monetary investments? The evaluators spent a great deal of time pondering that question and realized that the districts in Uganda were contiguous with Kampala, which enabled doctors in those districts to reach out to their better trained and better equipped colleagues in the nation's capital. In addition, Uganda made a greater investment in what Kruk called "active ingredients": vouchers for care, "mama kits" to offset the cost of care for women, a bigger health workforce, more extensive training and mentoring, and upgraded infrastructure.

One of the most important conclusions from the evaluation was that the program is too complicated. "There is no way this 28-point model will be replicated in the same way," said Kruk. "It's just too big." What the program should focus on, she said, are its active ingredients—the few things that made a significant difference when applied as a mutually reinforcing set of actions. In fact, one of the evaluations' recommendations was that the program should think in terms of health system packages, not isolated interventions. Core health system investments, she added, create a culture of competence. The evaluation also identified so-called last mile women— those who are isolated and have the hardest time getting to a health care facility. Another recommendation was that the program needs to commit to a duration of 5 years with a transition plan that clarifies the roles and responsibilities of partners and governments. Finally, the evaluation recommended that training is not enough. "We love capacity building and training," said Kruk. "That's something we know how to do. It's the backbone of global health assistance, but we don't think it's working well enough for the money spent, according to our findings."

In closing, Kruk said that one recommendation an evaluator should never make is to have more evaluation. Instead, the evaluation team noted the importance of treating the next phase of the project as a learning opportunity.

AVAHAN—REDUCING THE SPREAD OF HIV IN INDIA

The goal of the Bill & Melinda Gates Foundation's Avahan program was to demonstrate that it was possible to scale a program within target groups, with India chosen as the demonstration country because of the alarming rise of HIV in India and the inadequacy of that country's response to the epidemic. At the time, there were no adequate models for a large program aimed at women sex workers or men who have sex with men, said Padma Chandrasekaran, previously at the Bill & Melinda Gates Foundation and now a member of the executive committee of the Chennai Angels investment group. Nonetheless, there was no doubt at the foundation that the proposed interventions would lead to impact. The other key assumption was that responsibility for the program would eventually transition to the Indian government, because it was not feasible for any private foundation to fund the program indefinitely.

Because of the enormity of the problem and the lack of infrastructure in India, the foundation committed at least $200 million to the program, with 17 percent of the money going to capacity building. The program also committed 10 percent of funds to advocacy and policy change, because the environment in India was hostile toward HIV and high-risk groups. The implementation programs, said Chandrasekaran, were large and complex and included efforts to distribute treatments for sexually transmitted infections and community mobilization to get hidden populations into clinics.

The evaluation effort consisted of separate design and implementation teams with oversight provided by an evaluation advisory group. The design group developed a detailed question tree that aimed to measure the scale, coverage, quality, and cost of services; the impact of Avahan on the epidemic in India; and the program's cost-effectiveness. Initially, the intent was to use only program data, but the evaluators realized the necessity of using government data, too. Chandrasekaran noted that the availability of data was graduated across districts in India. For example, 4 districts had general population studies, while 29 districts had data from behavioral studies from the core high-risk groups.

Challenges included data collection among high-risk groups and getting data out for analysis, said Chandrasekaran. "Our evaluation grantees were international grantees, but they could not work in the country without local participatory institutions, and the local participatory institutions felt extremely possessive about the data that they had collected." The solution was to create incentives to encourage data sharing, including funding for workshops, training on how to write papers, and support for journal supplements. The result, said Chandrasekaran, was that once local institutions got their first publication out, data sharing with the international grantees became an easier proposition. In addition, all international grantees shared authorship with the local institutions that generated the data.

Chandrasekaran finished her presentation with a brief discussion of the program's scorecard. One positive point was the program included evaluation in its mission from the start, which allowed the design team to develop a clear theory of change, a clear theory of action, and a prospective design. The program was data rich, she said, and monitoring data was used to good effect. There was effective in-country evaluation capacity building, so much so that the Indian government conducted what Chandrasekaran characterized as a good, formal evaluation of its own HIV programs once the Avahan evaluation results were released. That evaluation, she added, was published in a premier journal and influenced the design of subsequent programs. "That was something that had never happened in the country before," she said. Finally, all of the foundation's data have been deposited in the public Harvard University Dataverse.

As far as what could have been done better, Chandrasekaran noted the evaluation was too costly and in retrospect could have been designed to be less expensive. In addition, the evaluation effort could have provided more up-front support for the government to collect surveillance data to better support the foundation's data collection. There were also several missed opportunities for implementing evaluations during rollout. As an example, she said that it would have been interesting to study what kind of drop-in centers work best with different target groups. "These are questions that could have had a short duration and provided cause-and-effect data," she said in closing.

EQUIP—EXPANDED QUALITY MANAGEMENT USING INFORMATION POWER

The EQUIP program, explained Tanya Marchant, an epidemiologist at the London School of Hygiene and Tropical Medicine, is designed to implement and evaluate the effect of a quality improvement intervention implemented at district, facility, and community levels designed to get all of the actors at the district level to work together to improve maternal and child health. The program targets demand for and supply of health care for mothers and newborns simultaneously, and what is most important about the program's approach, said Marchant, is that it "supports quality improvement with high-quality, locally generated data that is timely and available at regular periods."

Marchant noted that EQUIP is a small-scale project compared to the others being discussed at the workshop, but that it is a critical project nonetheless. The program operates in two districts in southern Tanzania and two districts in eastern Uganda. By relying on existing infrastructure organized within district-level health systems, EQUIP was able to engage with district health management teams, which in turn were able to support subdistrict, local quality improvement processes. The conceptual framework, Marchant explained, is built on the hypothesis that district-level health facilities are the best places to target quality improvement, but that communities are the best place to affect uptake of services.

One strength of this project is that it has continuous household and linked health facility survey data from all of the districts throughout the intervention period. The data are exported into report cards so information can be reported back to the facilities, communities, and districts simultaneously. "All three of these levels of actors have access to the same evidence, all of which is about them and their environment," explained Marchant, who added that the evidence is also fed back to the national level to foster engagement with the program.

The evaluation had four objectives: assess the effects of the intervention on the use and quality of service provision for maternal and newborn health; estimate the cost and cost-effectiveness of the intervention; assess the feasibility and acceptability of the intervention; and model the potential impact on mortality. While the continuous stream of data is key to the evaluation, contextual data is also important, and the program has a prospective contextual tracking process in place.

The evaluation has a quasi-experimental design that compares continuous household and health facility surveys in districts that participate in the EQUIP intervention to comparison districts that are not participating in the intervention in each country. The main difference between the intervention and comparison districts is that the intervention district has the quality management system with report cards generated from continuous survey data. The comparison districts receive a straightforward 100-page report annually that is a tabulation of indicators generated by the continuous survey. "I don't think it would be ethical to do such intensive data collection and not share anything with the comparison districts, but there is no facilitation," said Marchant. In response to a question about whether the EQUIP evaluation was an evaluation rather than a monitoring activity, Marchant said that it tested whether continuous surveying and providing feedback drives quality improvement more than just continuous surveying alone.

Expanding on the nature of the continuous surveys, Marchant said they are run in comparison and intervention districts for 30 months. They are based on an idea from the more traditional intermittent, large-scale perceptual surveys—such as DHS—that a rolling survey could have a sufficient sample size to report on a core set of indicators that the country was interested in at annual intervals. This would be accompanied by much smaller and more focused geographical analysis at more frequent intervals. One challenge to implementing this type of survey in a program such as EQUIP is that it requires a mechanism in place to support it over a 30-month period.

The household survey samples 10 clusters, with 30 households per cluster, from the entire district each month. The survey includes interviews with household heads, a household roster, and an interview with each woman age 13 to 49 about her health care and her fertility history, with a special module for any woman who had given birth in the last year. Marchant noted that the data can be aggregated for any number of consecutive months. Data collection also includes a complete census of all health care facilities in each district every 4 months with an assessment of service provision and in-depth interviews with midwives about the last birth they attended.

Every 4 months, the project team runs the data through an automated system that calculates indicators and creates the report cards for use in the intervention. Marchant noted that automation enables the project team to generate the report cards and go back into the field to provide feedback in 4–6 weeks. The report cards are discussed by staff and community members in scheduled meetings at the district health facilities to determine what the facility and the community can do to make improvements. These are run independently of the program. "EQUIP is there just to bring the groups together and give them high-quality, local information," Marchant said.

In the end, the EQUIP team found that continuous surveys are feasible to use and, if properly designed, can be managed with one data manager on each team who is supported from a distance. However, continuous surveys require continuous field work, so the team tried to avoid scheduling surveys during the rainy season or during the agricultural season. The use of personal digital assistants was incredibly important, Marchant said, because they boost data quality and control and because they enable automated data harvesting and analysis. It was also important to keep the questionnaire content up to date and internally consistent. In this case, there were few indicators of newborn health when EQUIP started, and it was important to add those indicators as the project proceeded.

One lesson the team learned regarding continuous feedback was that it required more facilitation than expected. "The people who are very good at motivating, who are committed, who are great community or facility members, are not necessarily the same people who are good at interpreting graphs and interpreting limitations and strengths of population household surveys or facility surveys," said Marchant.

Responding to a question about the cost of continuous surveying, she said that her team budgets $20 per household, and in Tanzania the cost was $17 per household or $7,200 per district for the entire study period. Another participant noted that this is an expensive proposition given that Tanzania spends $30 per capita annually on health services.

OTHER TOPICS RAISED IN DISCUSSION

Kruk pointed out that every evaluation creates opportunity costs. Evaluators therefore need to be very honest with themselves about the value they are adding to an initiative. However, evaluations also can help initiatives develop theories of change that can greatly increase the effectiveness of an initiative, though such theories are also heavily dependent on context.

Chandrasekaran also addressed costs, noting that the Avahan program spent about 10 percent on evaluation on the advice of an independent design group. However, a learning process reduced costs of specific evaluation components over time. Also, aspects of the evaluation represented extremely good investments, she said, because of their effects on the program.

Finally, Marchant and Kruk both commented on the fact that program implementers often do not have a good understanding of how an intervention is supposed to work and what it is supposed to achieve, partly because of a lack of communication and partly because a program can evolve over time. Evaluations can help interventions "have clarity about what you are and how you get to where you're going," said Marchant. Granted, a logic model can change over time, sometimes in response to an evaluation, but part of an evaluation is to codify what is supposed to be happening and what is actually happening.

11

Using Evaluation Findings and Communicating Key Messages

Important Points Made by the Speakers

- Succinct reports, transparency of processes and findings, and wide dissemination can increase the use of evaluation results.
- Developing a communications plan when designing an evaluation can increase the use of findings.
- Putting findings and recommendations into context for local governments and other local stakeholders can strengthen programs on the ground.
- Evaluation results can be especially useful if synthesized and disseminated through structured forums at the country level.

In this session, the workshop addressed issues related to the complexity of the diverse uses and audiences for large-scale evaluations and the importance of matching the message, the messenger, and the audience. Panelists also spoke about the challenges associated with tracking the use of large-scale evaluation findings.

"Our assumption," said moderator Sir George Alleyne, chancellor of the University of the West Indies, in introducing the panel, "is that evaluation findings are useful, but being useful is not the same thing as being used." It is incumbent, then, for evaluators to promote and propose mechanisms to ensure that evaluation findings are used. "I think it is unjust and unfair not to make maximum use of evaluation findings," he stated.

THE U.S. PRESIDENT'S MALARIA INITIATIVE

Bernard Nahlen, deputy coordinator of the PMI, began the panel presentation by recounting the genesis of the PMI, which was launched in mid-2005 with an initial congressional authorization of $1.2 billion over 5 years. A response to criticism of the U.S. Malaria Program administered by USAID, the PMI was intended to target 15 high-burden countries in Africa. The main criticism of that program was that, while it conducted good research and generated many documents, there was no evidence that the program was doing anything to turn the tide against the rising burden of malaria in these high-burden countries. Another criticism was that the U.S. part of the program relied too heavily on a social marketing model and that it lacked any effort to develop capacity for countries to do indoor residual spraying or to distribute mosquito nets.

As authorized by Congress, PMI's funds would come through USAID, with CDC the U.S. government's main implementing agency. The PMI, in contrast to PEPFAR, was not "afflicted with many earmarks and targets," Nahlen said. The PMI was designed to have a small personnel footprint, with two resident advisors, one hired by USAID and the other by CDC, operating out of each in-country USAID health office. Each office also employed one or two local staff to help manage the program. By mid-2006, the PMI was operating in three countries; six more came online in 2007; and by 2008 the effort was operational in all 15 countries in Africa.

The program started with a clear business model, strong leadership in the person of retired admiral Tim Ziemer, and a country-level Malaria Operational Planning Process. The program was established with the provision for yearly reviews, in which program teams visited each country to work with the national programs to develop an understanding of the status of each program at that time. The 15 countries were chosen in part because they had additional globally funded malaria grants from organizations such as the Global Fund, the World Bank, and other funders working in the malaria space. To counter the criticism that USAID country offices had too much autonomy in administering program funds, the PMI had a clear mandate with targets and defined interventions that would be delivered. These mandates, said Nahlen, created some initial pushback from USAID staff and from CDC.

The PMI functions as a learning environment, Nahlen noted, in which program staff appear to be willing to try different approaches and learn from experience. In that context, the PMI decided to launch an evaluation, even though it was not mandated by Congress, and ask for actionable recommendations. In the end, the evaluators made 10 recommendations, 5 on the technical side and 5 on the policy and programmatic side. To disseminate the report and its recommendations, Nahlen used an interagency advisory group comprising representatives of CDC, the National Institutes of Health (NIH), and the Office of Global Health in the Department of Health and Human Services; the Department of Defense; the Department of State; the Office of Management and Budget; and the Peace Corps. His office also posted the report on its website, sent an e-card to 27,500 USAID users, and distributed the report at the country level through its resident in-country advisors.

The report generated many responses, said Nahlen. Congress responded to the report's recommendations with an increase in funding that has enabled the PMI to expand into four additional African countries and initiate a program in the Mekong Delta region. The report also recommended that the PMI increase its personnel footprint, particularly as it moved into countries such as Nigeria and the Democratic Republic of the Congo. Adding highly qualified local staff, the PMI not only has built capacity in these countries but also has created stability in the local programs.

Another recommendation called for the PMI to increase the flow of money through local government programs, but there was the concern about the money getting commodities to the people in need. Nahlen's group has assessed this situation and found that of the 19 African countries, more money is now flowing through local ministries of health and the national control programs in 14 countries. In three countries—Madagascar, Mali, and Zimbabwe—U.S. government restrictions prohibit direct funding. As a final note, Nahlen said that in response to a recommendation, the PMI has hired an operational research coordinator to establish a research framework and set priorities. Talks are ongoing with WHO and other funders to ensure that the PMI's operational research agenda complements what others are doing.

ROADS TO A HEALTHY FUTURE

The focus of the Roads to a Healthy Future program, which is funded by PEPFAR through USAID, is to address HIV and health issues along transport corridors and to examine the structural drivers of the spread of HIV, explained Dorothy Muroki, project director of the program. Many aspects of the PEPFAR evaluation report, she said, were relevant to strengthening the Roads to a Healthy Future program; in particular, she discussed two key examples of recommendations resulting in action.

In the summary findings for HIV prevention, the evaluation recognized that interventions targeted at prevention of sexual transmission, including biomedical, behavioral, and structural interventions, are all critical components of a balanced and comprehensive prevention portfolio. The report also recognized that, within PEPFAR, less program monitoring data and vigorous research evidence were available on these interventions, particularly behavioral and structural interventions, as compared with the other biomedical interventions such as preventing mother-to-child transmission. "As an implementer, this for me was a stark reminder that gaps in the evidence base around behavioral and structural interventions persisted within my own program, but also across the public health fraternity," Muroki explained. Moreover, she and her team realized that this gap in the evidence base was undermining support for these two critical elements of balanced programming because there was not enough evidence proving that the program's behavioral and structural interventions were working.

In response, one of the steps she and her colleagues took was to examine the association between improved economic status of households and use of health services. "What we are going to do with the data is strengthen our own programming, and we'll package it for use by host governments and other stakeholders," Muroki said. She added that these data have generated interest in Rwanda, Tanzania, and Zambia, the three countries where her team is finalizing the study.

The second example of the usefulness of the PEPFAR evaluation that she discussed involves reexamining gender-based programming in the Roads to a Healthy Future project. Since 2005 the program had been promoting gender equity in decision making at more than 65 sites along the transport corridors, but the evaluation led her team to examine whether its local partners had the skills and tools to sustain this work, or if gender expertise was instead embedded solely within its team members. "We realized that it was important for us to look at strengthening and locally implementing partners so that they would be able to address gender issues, which was very critical for program success over the long term," Muroki said. As a result, she has tapped into her organization's technical expertise on gender issues to support local community partners' efforts to build expertise in this area, which she said has had a positive impact on gender programming.

Addressing the issue of communication, Muroki said, "my perspective is that the evaluation findings could be even more useful if synthesized and disseminated through structured forums at the country level. For me the synthesis issue is critical because the [evaluation] reports are voluminous, and truth be told, is an implementer going to read the volumes? Most likely not. So having ways and means of synthesizing the information and using structured forums to be able to disseminate the information is important." She also suggested that findings and recommendations should be put into context for local governments so evaluation findings can be used to strengthen programs on the ground. In closing, she wondered if opportunities exist for there to be more collaboration between collaborative evaluations run by different funders working on similar programs within individual countries, particularly with regard to disseminating findings. "This could create synergies that would probably push the use of the findings," said Muroki. "With information overload being an ever-present challenge in our world today, I think the public health evaluation community must engage audiences in ways that cut through their own clutter, whether we're thinking of individuals or of organizations and institutions. Identifying and developing strategies to make this information easier to access, digest, and act upon, for me, is a critical step for consideration going forward."

THE SOUTH AFRICAN PERSPECTIVE ON INFLUENCING POLICY AND PERFORMANCE

In November 2011, South Africa approved a National Evaluation Policy that created the Department of Performance Monitoring and Evaluation in the Office of the President. The goal of this act was to determine if services being delivered in South Africa were benefitting people on the ground. To date, said Ian Goldman, head of evaluation and research in the department, 38 evaluations have looked at several billion dollars' worth of government programs. Each evaluation is focused on utilization—are the services offered by a program being utilized on the ground—and therefore emphasizes learning. One challenge that Goldman and his colleagues face is getting individual departments to take ownership of these evaluations, and his team is addressing this challenge by getting departments to determine what they want to evaluate.

Once an evaluation is completed, Goldman's team creates an improvement plan, which will be monitored for 2 years to determine if the evaluations trigger action by the departments. Complementing this effort is a training program on evidence-based policy making for permanent secretaries, senior management teams, and members of the South African parliament. To incentivize departments to suggest evaluation topics, beyond the desire to improve performance, Goldman's office pays for 50 percent of an evaluation. "We focus on the process as much as the product because a good product with poor process will not be used," he said. Even then, he acknowledges, capacity in South Africa is limited, so his office is strategic about the evaluations it conducts and is limiting its initial efforts to 15 priority evaluations annually.

To promote independence the evaluations are undertaken by service providers, with input from a steering committee representing key stakeholders. To boost the quality of the evaluations, Goldman's office has developed evaluation standards, competency training, and a peer review committee. His team also conducts a quality assessment within a month after an evaluation is completed based on these standards. In addition, his department is conducting an "evaluation of evaluations" to see whether the work it has done is having an impact.

Communication is emphasized, Goldman said, and his office has developed a guideline that all reports should have a 1-page policy summary, a 5-page executive summary, and a body of the report that does not exceed 25 pages. Transparency is also key, so every report is posted to the department website along with a quality assessment, improvement plan, and progress reports, enabling the public to track what is happening. One of South Africa's goals is to get all countries to use the same standardized terminology when it conducts evaluations so the countries can more easily learn from each other's experiences.

COMMUNICATING RESULTS FROM THE PEPFAR EVALUATION

When the IOM does a consensus study, explained Kimberly Scott, who was one of the study co-directors for the IOM's PEPFAR evaluation, it requires that a communications and dissemination plan be developed before the study is approved. In the case of the IOM evaluation of PEPFAR, dissemination and communication activities were included in the evaluation contract. Scott noted that the audience for the PEPFAR evaluation was quite diverse, including Congress, the Department of State, the Office of the Global AIDS Coordinator, the PEPFAR implementation agencies, others involved in national and global responses to HIV, and the general public.

Dissemination focused on three types of activities. One was issuing a variety of reports and report products such as the ones discussed at the workshop. In addition to the main report, which is available in hard copy and free in electronic format, the IOM prepared a 20-page executive summary that outlined the 13 recommendations from the evaluation and a 4-page policy brief. The IOM staff and committee members also engaged in a large number of in-person briefings, including a pre-release briefing for the Office of the Global AIDS Coordinator and its director, Ambassador Eric Goosby. Because the study was mandated by Congress, the IOM staff held briefings for congressional staff and for the committees of jurisdiction, as well as for several other committees that were interested and requested separate briefings.

Scott said that one of the most important types of briefing was to the PEPFAR implementing agencies and the technical staff of those agencies. An interesting characteristic was that the staff of those agencies established the agenda for the briefings, giving staff the opportunity to pick the technical areas that were most relevant to them and to ask about details with some specificity. This briefing also gave staff at the implementing agencies opportunities to talk with the IOM staff and committee members about the technical details that went into the recommendations so that they might actually develop implementation plans for those recommendations. "Part of what we learned after we issued the report was that Ambassador Goosby required a written response from all of the implementation agencies to the report's findings and recommendations," said Scott. "And while that wasn't going to be for public distribution, that was one tool that he was using to be able to break down and digest what was relevant in the report, to talk about it with the implementation agencies and their technical staff, and to discuss with them how they were going to use the report."

The IOM also did two public briefings, one when it released the report and another planned strategically for several months after the report's release. "We knew that people would need time to be able to digest the information in the report and to be able to have some meaningful dialog," Scott explained. Both of the public briefings were webcast globally and an effort was made to encourage country-level participation, including participation in the briefing in person by representatives from Ghana, Kenya, Mali, and Tanzania. The IOM committee members and staff have also been invited to participate in events, including one focused on funders in the HIV/AIDS realm that allowed the IOM staff to educate donors about some of the significant issues in the report, and another for the UNAIDS Monitoring and Evaluation Reference Group meeting. The evaluation was also presented and discussed at scientific meetings, at the Consortium for Universities for Global Health Annual Conference, where committee members and staff did presentations on the methods and the findings, and at the Annual Qualitative Research for Health Conference.

In addition, the committee chair wrote an editorial for the *Lancet*, and there were blogs about the evaluation from, for example, the Center for Strategic and International Development and the Center for Global Development. For the project webpage, the IOM created a brief quiz that focused on disease education and provided a global epidemiological perspective as well as a more in-depth interactive experience. This interactive experience has two functions, Scott explained. First, it describes what PEPFAR does in terms of the types of services it provides; second, it illustrates what an experience might be in a PEPFAR country in trying to access prevention, treatment, or care services.

The IOM has a limited ability to track the use of its findings and recommendations, but some metrics are available, such as new legislation or changes in funding. The IOM also scans relevant websites and news outlets to track use of the report, and study staff have periodic opportunities to follow up with implementing agencies to find out how reports are being used and to get feedback. For example, said Scott, "We have gotten some very specific feedback that some technical areas will now be changing their indicators to do outcome measurement as opposed to outputs, and to start to do some age disaggregation of data." Finally, the IOM has enough flexibility to link continued activities with work it has done in the past, as in the case of this workshop.

OTHER TOPICS RAISED IN DISCUSSION

The conversation during the discussion session focused on several broad issues in the communication and use of evaluation findings, including the diversity of audiences, the budget for dissemination, the independence of evaluators, the responsibility for dissemination, and the transparency of evidence.

Muroki noted that different participants in an evaluation have different needs, incentives, and interests, and as a result they can have different audiences in mind when preparing an evaluation. Aspects of communication and dissemination need to be treated from the beginning with the same seriousness as the technical aspects of an evaluation, she said.

With regard to funding, Nahlen said that his budget was $500,000, which was "very good value for money" with a program that spends hundreds of millions of dollars annually. He also said that his office at the PMI uses a tracking sheet for its 10 primary recommendations that it updates regularly. Goldman said that his department's evaluations cost between $150,000 and $400,000 each. He said his organization requires that departments produce a management response when an evaluation is produced and publicly released. This is used to create an improvement plan that is then tracked. However, dissemination is still "embryonic," he said, with more work needed on targeted marketing.

With regard to the budget specifically for dissemination, Scott noted that in general the IOM dissemination represents a relatively small part of overall project budgets. Aspects of dissemination are part of the core activities of the IOM studies, said Scott, but many extra activities depend on volunteer time from staff and committee members.

Nahlen emphasized the importance of producing actionable recommendations for an evaluation to have impact. Recommendations that are self-evident or "nice to know" are hard to implement by the audiences of an evaluation. The question of the independence of program evaluators was also raised during the discussion. As Nahlen pointed out, evaluators can sometimes be so independent that their recommendations are not actionable because they are too separated from an initiative. At the same time, a balance is necessary to avoid conflicts of interest.

The audiences for an evaluation often have a shared responsibility in not only implementing but tracking and disseminating the recommendations of an evaluation, several panel members noted. "Dissemination is not disseminating to them," said Goldman. "They're part of the process." As

Scott added, "It is often up to the sponsor to determine what will happen in terms of dissemination."

Making disseminations public—as well as the data on which they are based—can have the effect of increasing implementation, Goldman added. Such transparency can be difficult, but it can help make a program a partner in an evaluation of that program. Goldman raised the point that many evaluations essentially amount to technical experts from northern countries telling program managers in southern countries what to do differently. The real issue is how evaluations can contribute to a change process through partnerships, he said.

12

Envisioning a Future for Evaluation

> **Important Points Made by the Speakers**
> - It is advantageous to introduce evaluative thinking at the beginning of a project.
> - Theories of change are important and can evolve over time as people's understanding of how programs work changes.
> - Instead of "did it work or not," more relevant and useful questions for evaluation are "What aspects worked, what aspects worked less well, what can be scaled up, what could be strengthened, and what can be sustained?"
> - Bringing about local change in local places requires an ecology of evidence, with knowledge translated for use and learning in real time.
> - Strong evaluations require an investment of resources, time, commitment, trust, and strong relationships.

On the final afternoon of the workshop, two experienced evaluators commented on their ideas for how to design a hypothetical evaluation of a fictitious global initiative that embodied many of the characteristics of the large, complex, multidisciplinary, global interventions that were the focus of the workshop. The idea behind the session, noted moderator Elliot Stern, emeritus professor of evaluation research at Lancaster University and visiting professor at Bristol University, was to think through some of the various designs, methods, and ideas that had been examined and discussed in this workshop.

Stern began the session by providing some details from the description of the fictitious initiative given to the evaluators. The objective of the initiative is to improve safe, reliable, and sustainable access to clean water in the Pacific Andean region. Three partner countries—Chile, Ecuador, and Peru—will select priority outcomes and develop and implement a portfolio of activities and interventions to achieve those outcomes. Funding of $3.4 billion is to be provided cooperatively by Fundación María Elena, a fictitious philanthropic foundation described as newly established by a wealthy South American banker, USAID, and the Canadian International Development Agency, with 10 percent of funding from locally sourced assets in each partner country. During a 1-year planning phase, a stakeholder coalition is to set priorities among such outcomes as improved health and well-being, environmental improvements, better water systems, improved public awareness, and reduced violence and crime due to water disputes. The coalition is also to assess needs, capacity, and current efforts; select a country portfolio of infrastructure investments and interventions; develop a sustainability plan; and develop a data collection plan.

During the 3-year implementation phase, the initiative's components could include, for example, building infrastructure for water systems; implementing technologies for water and sanitation services at the community and household level; developing and installing technologies for monitoring water quality; education campaigns; and behavior change interventions. A subsequent 4-year extension phase could involve another planning and prioritization process and an increase in the local resource matching requirement to 25 percent. A long-term sustainability phase could follow the 8-year intervention.

The premise presented to the panelists, explained Stern, was that the funders have requested an evaluation for the first 4 years of the initiative—a planning year followed by an initial 3-year implementation phase. The evaluation budget will be approximately $3 million. The main objectives of the evaluation would be to assess the effects of the initiative on the availability of and safe access to clean water and on other priority outcomes selected by partner countries, to assess the operational performance of the initiative, and to inform the planning and implementation of the extension and long-term phases. Additional evaluation aims might include assessments of each country's process for prioritization and planning, local match requirements for funding, multisectoral participation, planning for sustainability, and the potential to adapt the model for other regions, such as Central America or East Africa.

FRAMING THE EVALUATION

Water issues address very specific health problems and have a major impact on health inequities, and this hypothetical initiative has "aspirations written all over it" but without specificity on how to get there, said Sanjeev Sridharan, director of the Evaluation Centre for Complex Health Interventions at Li Ka Shing Knowledge Institute at St. Michaels Hospital. But that is not unusual. "That is the nature of 90 percent of the interventions I evaluate," said Sridharan. Indeed, a lack of specificity provides an opportunity to introduce evaluative thinking at the beginning of a project rather than the end, but he argued against spending excessive time thinking about the best design at the beginning of a project, when the project is still being developed. Large-scale complex programs inevitably have designs never implemented before, but they have components that are familiar. The package of familiar components and how they coalesce is what makes an intervention complex. This project, he said, "is begging for some developmental evaluation, where the evaluation team itself participates in the development of an intervention."

Charlotte Watts, head of the Social and Mathematical Epidemiology Group and founding director of the Gender, Violence, and Health Centre in the Department for Global Health and Development at the London School of Hygiene and Tropical Medicine, agreed, suggesting that national researchers from the countries where the intervention will take place should be part of the evaluation from the very beginning to embed the element of capacity building in to the evaluation. Success takes time, and engaging stakeholders on the ground is a good way to get moving in the right direction. Evaluators need to move away from the idea of "best design." Interventions and designs need to be treated as portfolios from which new knowledge can emerge.

But great plans do not equal great implementation. Implementations need structures and support systems to produce improved health and well-being, Sridharan observed. He was taught, as an evaluator, to pretend that interventions are well formed from the beginning, but after 20 years of experience he has yet to find a well-formed intervention on day 1. "Interventions are complex, they're dynamic, they change over time. In fact, they should be—that's what learning implies."

Sridharan also pointed out that evaluators need to think through timelines early on to be realistic with funders and others about what results evaluations can deliver and when. People in communities have been thinking about the problems they face for a very long time, yet administrators can want results from an evaluation in very short time periods. During the discussion period, Watts also pointed out that such time pressures can undermine research in many ways. Evaluators need time to think and pre-test an approach if they are to deliver a rigorous evaluation, but funders can overlook this need. "The risk is that we say something doesn't work when actually it just hasn't had the time to kick in and have an effect."

Watts noted that it is important to understand the desired outputs that are to be achievements of the evaluation, and that while in this scenario there are specific and multiple objectives, there are also broader public good elements that can often accompany large-scale evaluations. These can include informed, intelligent intervention delivery; an increasing capacity for strengthened networks and ownership of programs with nationally led evaluation and research; and the use of monitoring and evaluation data by program staff and practitioners.

Watts was struck by the three categorizations of purpose of evaluation stated earlier in the workshop by Chris Witty: (1) assurance to the pay masters who are funding the evaluation; (2) cost correction, which may be addressed more toward good management by improving programs by learning and thinking how we use evaluation approaches to learn by doing versus evaluation; and (3) impact evaluation. Watts queried as to whether these evaluation purposes are mutually exclusive because she stated that most evaluations should be striving to accomplish all three. In the end, stated Watts, understanding that program effectiveness cannot be reduced to answering a closed-ended question about whether "it worked"—an evaluator translating evaluation findings as a simple "this works or it does not work"—can be interpreted as a commentary on the life work of the implementer and is not a good start to a working relationship. Often people are implementing combinations of programs that have some proven elements that work, so how do you actually make sure that as well as answering the questions the donors want answered, you also think about the questions that programs really want you to answer, and explicitly include that in your evaluation design? Perhaps the evaluation questions should be more nuanced: Can you do it at scale? Can you do it with this population? Can you sustain it? To Watts, this provides a greater space for the framing of questions, the evaluation design, and for partnership between evaluators and program staff.

Both evaluators emphasized the critical importance of understanding contextual factors for the evaluation. The relationship between context and the desired outcomes is important for intervention and evaluation designs. Sridharan noted it is best to bring the knowledge of context in at the start, but reminded the audience that we have to be evolving and adapting over time. He noted that evaluations tend to be based on the premise that the world is understood, but this is not the case. Knowledge of context therefore needs to continually inform evaluations so they can evolve over time.

Furthermore, Sridharan noted that for this intervention, paying attention to interdependences will be critical, given the variations in geography, the presence of extractive industries, and possible disputes. The countries in which the interventions are being implemented have various tensions and problems, and because water does not necessarily follow national boundaries context extends to surrounding countries such as Argentina and Bolivia that are inevitably going to be involved as well. Ongoing agreements will be a crucial factor in the planning. Sridharan said that a cooperative funding stream can produce powerful partnerships, but a mechanism is needed to develop these partnerships. The presence of a large amount of funding can actually be an impediment to developing partnerships. The planning process will also need to pay attention to needs, capacities, infrastructure, local assets, implementation, political power, and project portfolios.

Independence

In response to a question from Stern about whether evaluators should stay strictly independent throughout an evaluation, Sridharan argued for a more nuanced position. Sridharan pointed out that most evaluators do not work directly in program settings. He also pointed out that program staff are generally among the most critical observers of their programs. It does not take a faraway researcher to be objective about a program. "That's not fair, and it's condescending. More and more, these folks are quite self-critical." Degrees of independence can be approached in phases. Early in a project, an evaluator may be able to provide valuable input to program staff as they design or modify an intervention. After this developmental phase, evaluators may need to achieve more independence from a program to deliver unbiased results, even if that means altering a relationship over time. Much of the time, a workshop participant pointed out, the implementer and the evaluator is the same person. As Stern added, it may be possible to have different people involved in different evaluation phases to obtain the appropriate levels of independence.

In a later discussion Stern noted that many of the words used in discussing evaluations—such as *impartial*, *objective*, *bias*, *engagement*, *empowerment*, *subjectivity*, and *intersubjectivity*—have strong histories and deserve much more attention and thought in evaluations than simply "are they independent or not."

BUILDING AN ECOLOGY OF EVIDENCE

The implementation of an intervention is a journey that begins with a theory of change. This theory in turn draws on an evidence base derived from prior journeys. The idea that global health initiatives are often a thumbs up or thumbs down after just a few years is nonsensical, noted Sridharan. Learning frameworks and pathways of influence are essential.

The theory of change will evolve over time and for that matter, theories of change can be subjected to experiments and quasi-experiments to formalize the learning process. "For learning you need explicit learning structures, and I don't think we often plan for that." By embedding evaluations in complex interventions, the evaluation can help improve the intervention, which means in essence that the evaluation is itself evaluated. Sridharan said that he was not opposed to traditional design and measuring impacts. "At the end you have to be saying was this a good investment?" But people rarely go back and think about what they have learned from an evaluation about an intervention. Revisiting evaluation methods annually helps inform both programming and continued evaluation, a point with which both Watts and Sridharan agreed. This process makes it easier to identify what to focus on, where to drill down on certain points, and how to collect final evaluation data. It also can contribute to the establishment of systems to encourage routine collection and use of monitoring data by programs. Monitoring systems and small nested studies could be used to troubleshoot and support the good management of programming.

Besides clarifying a theory of change, Sridharan recommended paying attention to contextual mechanisms, referring back to the earlier presentation on realist evaluation. How are activities controlled? Can the desired interventions really solve the problems that exist? How long will it take for impacts to appear, and what metrics will be used to measure those impacts? Do the metrics provide incentives to stay true to the intervention? What unintended consequences could occur? How does the plan address heterogeneous contexts? How are the aspects of an intervention aligned?

Watts supported spending time at the beginning of a project to develop a theory of change. A theory of change makes it possible to revisit design plans, frame data collection and feedback, and replicate interventions in other settings. In contrast, she was unenthusiastic about the logical framework approach, which she judged to be difficult to use, especially with low literacy populations or evaluation staff. She recommended trying to keep materials relatively straightforward and usable by program staff and researchers. She challenged participants to be more creative about using evaluation frameworks as a programming and monitoring tool. She was also enthusiastic about the prospects of using smartphones or other new technologies to facilitate rapid collection of output data. Looping that feedback into programs could be very powerful.

The measurement of impacts is a long-term process, said Sridharan, not a one-shot method. Also, a knowledge base is developed for local interventions, not just for people or policy makers in faraway cities. For this reason, an evidence base is not enough. To bring about change in local places, an ecology of evidence is needed. A single store of evidence is not sufficient to bring about change. Program theory is also insufficient, in part because of the inevitable uncertainties in a program theory. Knowledge also needs to be translated for use in real time. "Far too often, our evaluation methodologies are grand reports that are not read by the people whose lives they're trying to improve," said Sridharan. "Capacity building is central, because it's not the grand outsider who's going to bring about a change."

Achieving Multiple Evaluation Aims

Evaluations of large-scale, complex, multi-national initiatives typically seek to achieve multiple objectives, said Watts. In pursuing these multiple goals, evaluators need to walk a tightrope, she continued. They need to provide assurances to funders that are specified in the terms of reference regarding rigorous evaluation of intervention impacts and cost-effectiveness. They may want to derive programmatic lessons about how to scale up effective interventions in other settings and the resources required to do that. They also may want to produce shared open datasets that are amenable for further analyses. In addition, they may aim to increase capacity for locally led evaluation and for use of monitoring and evaluation data by program staff. All of these tasks overlap said Watts. "These are things that most evaluations should be striving to do."

Considerations for Evaluation Design and Methods

When thinking about the design for this complex intervention, there are some things to keep in mind, said Watts. To balance all of the different demands and multiple evaluation aims, there is a need to really try to make the proposed evaluation a prospective, mixed methods study conducted by a multidisciplinary team. Considerations for the design are to include economic evaluation in the methods and to carefully consider the sampling frame because the groups who are most vulnerable are where we want to see whether the change is occurring—samplings linked to that will need a lot of thought. All countries should be included, with intervention and control communities in each country and, ideally, some sort of randomization. This may not always be possible, but it deserves energy and creative thinking—many interventions can be designed to include some element of randomness from which important information can be learned. For example, a program can be rolled out in a staggered way with a random allocation of where interventions start. To this, Stern added that the appropriateness of randomized controlled trials depends on the questions being asked. For example, trials may not be appropriate for investigations of whether a particular program can be scaled up or customized for a particular setting.

Watts raised some questions about the best ways to use mixed methods in order to optimize the quantitative, qualitative, and economic evaluation components. She asked, How can we ensure that mixed methods are indeed mixed and not parallel? In a way, when we're doing large evaluations we have a bit of an engine that's moving. However, qualitative work can be proactively and flexibly nested into quantitative studies by embedding researchers into the program to enable course corrections and provision of timely data. These efforts can be low cost, influential, and are appreciated by programs on the ground. Watts challenged workshop participants to think about the best way to incorporate economic questions and questions about resource use into mixed methods models. Evaluations need to strive to achieve key design elements, Watts continued.

In addition to course correction over time, evaluations can also assess the delivery of combinations of "proven packages" at scale, where many different factors determine success or may derail or hinder success. The challenges of program delivery need to be acknowledged, she said, including similarities and differences between settings and the expertise of program staff. Interventions are complex, they have to be adaptive, and research is needed to support that adaptation. Reasonable targets make it possible to work backwards to measures of potentially small effect sizes over limited time frames. "These sorts of elements are really important to think through at the start and to have explicit in your design," said Watts. In this process, it is important to develop a clear sense of the planned delivery chain and potential bottlenecks. There will be variations in coverage and impact, which requires getting good measures of intervention exposure and proxies of success over time.

Sridharan concurred about the need to develop measures of success, noting that these will have to evolve over time. If they do not, an evaluation risks finding what it set out to find or reporting no impact when the impacts are different than expected.

Sridharan also observed that this example is a long-term initiative by the description, and sustainability is an explicit goal. No one would expect health in Chile or Peru to change dramatically in 1 or 2 years, he stated, yet the evaluations are going to at least begin during those years. Even $3.4 billion projects need to be scaled up and generalized if they are to have the effect that is ultimately intended. Evaluators have not done a good enough job of examining the concept of generalization in a complex and contextual world, said Sridharan. Initial evaluations therefore have to recognize that evaluations will continue into the longer term and build the capacity for those longer-term evaluations. In this way, dynamic and evolving evaluations can contribute to continual improvements. Stern added that developing capacity extends not only to skills and networks but to developing data capacity. Some parts of a program may even need to be delayed to put in place a monitoring system that will allow subsequent analysis.

Watts also noted that a process of sharing and explaining context and programmatic experience as part of the evaluation design is important for political buy-in to attempt introduction of the intervention into different settings, as well as for facilitating bidirectional learning for evaluators and researchers to generate research questions and document evidence of success or effectiveness. Based on her experiences doing a 10-country study on violence against women, Watts cited the importance of building trust and strong working relationships. For the hypothetical case, she said that she would want to have annual face-to-face meetings along with online communications and debate. These communications should bring program staff together with national and international evaluators, creating a two-way learning process that can motivate both sides. Together, this group could ask what worked well, what worked less well, how to address bottlenecks, and how to share lessons and strengthen programming. Cross-disciplinary, research-practitioner discussions could support a common agenda of making evaluations work to help interventions achieve their greatest impact and deliver programs efficiently.

CAPACITY BUILDING FOR FUTURE EVALUATORS

Capacity building for future evaluators and researchers was raised during the discussion during this session. In thinking about how best to train students to formulate relevant, strategic, and important questions before focusing an evaluation's design, Sridharan emphasized the importance of humility. People may be trained to use sophisticated evaluation tools, but they may limit the solution space before bringing those tools to bear on a problem. "The first lesson of solution space is to work with communities, be humble, go home and reflect on these issues." Watts agreed with the need for humility, especially in complex interventions where evaluators need to spend a lot of time understanding the intricacies of a program, especially given that research methods can be blunt tools. Nevertheless, researchers need to be objective and do good science, even as they are invested in the programs they are evaluating. "You care, but the way that you care is by wanting to learn what actually works." Programs need to learn, and evaluators can help them do so by asking the right questions and having strong research designs.

Rachel Nugent, University of Washington, noted that many students have become interested in what is variously termed *implementation science* or *program science*. Funding agencies such as NIH also are becoming interested and are beginning to fund this approach. Stern said that his reading of implementation science is that it remains based on randomization and controlled experiments. But many knowledge gaps exist in such areas as how programs are implemented, how stakeholders are engaged, and what kind of preplanning needs to take place. Watts pointed out that implementation science involves embedding research to improve programs, which resonates strongly with the approach she has been advocating.

Watts observed more generally that strong evaluations pose a challenge for current public health models of evaluation training and development. "Are the models of public health evaluation that we teach our students broad and flexible enough? We teach them the essence of good evaluation design and randomized controlled trials. [But] as people go into their specializations, are we supporting them to learn how to work effectively as researchers with program? Are we supporting them to be able to bring together different disciplines?... If that skill gets developed, then this sort of intervention model will become more feasible." Watts observed that in the incentive structures evaluators face, they are rewarded for publishable results based on rigorous designs. When asked to look at issues that are complicated and murky, they may worry about the risks to their careers. The challenge is to create incentives for more difficult evaluations so researchers do not shy away from such work. Strong evaluations require resources, commitment, investments, trust, and strong relationships, Watts concluded, but they can be tremendously beneficial for public health.

References

Action to Control Cardiovascular Risk in Diabetes Study Group, H. C. Gerstein, M. E. Miller, R. P. Byington, D. C. Goff, Jr., J. T. Bigger, J. B. Buse, W. C. Cushman, S. Genuth, F. Ismail-Beigi, R. H. Grimm, Jr., J. L. Probstfield, D. G. Simons-Morton, and W. T. Friedewald. 2008. Effects of intensive glucose lowering in type 2 diabetes. *New England Journal of Medicine* 358(24):2545–2559.

Berk, R. A., and P. H. Rossi. 1999. *Thinking about program evaluation 2*. Thousand Oaks, CA: Sage Publications, Inc.

BetterEvaluation. 2014. *BetterEvaluation: Sharing information to improve evaluation*. http://betterevaluation.org (accessed April 7, 2014).

Carugi, C. 2014. *Panel 4: Analyzing data using triangulation in a mixed methods evaluation to reach overall findings, conclusions, and recommendations*. Paper presented at the Board on Global Health Workshop, Evaluation Methods for Large-Scale, Complex, Multi-National Global Health Initiatives, London, United Kingdom, Wellcome Trust, April 17.

Goodman, C. 2014. *Panel 2: Developing the evaluation design and methodological approaches*. Paper presented at the Board on Global Health Workshop, Evaluation Methods for Large-Scale, Complex, Multi-National Global Health Initiatives, London, United Kingdom, Wellcome Trust, April 17.

IOM (Institute of Medicine). 2013. *Evaluation of PEPFAR*. Washington, DC: The National Academies Press.

IOM and NRC (National Research Council). 2010. *Strategic approach to the evaluation of programs implemented under the Tom Lantos and Henry J. Hyde U.S. Global Leadership Against HIV/AIDS, Tuberculosis, and Malaria Reauthorization Act of 2008*. Washington, DC: The National Academies Press.

Lauer, M. S., and R. B. D'Agostino. 2013. The randomized registry trial—the next disruptive technology in clinical research? *New England Journal of Medicine* 369(17):1579–1581.

Leeuw, F., and J. Vaessen. 2009. *Impact evaluations and development: NONIE guidance on impact evaluation*. Washington, DC: Network of Networks on Impact Evaluation (NONIE).

Patton, M. P. 2002. *Qualitative research and evaluation methods.* Thousand Oaks, CA: Sage Publications, Inc.

Pawson, R. 2013. *The science of evaluation: A realist manifesto.* London: Sage.

Rogers, P. J. 2008. Using programme theory to evaluate complicated and complex aspects of interventions. *Evaluation* 14(1):29–48.

Rossi, P. H., M. W. Lipsey, and H. E. Freeman. 2004. *Evaluation: A systematic approach.* Thousand Oaks, CA: Sage Publications, Inc.

Royse, D., B. A. Thyer, and D. K. Padgett. 2009. *Program evaluation: An introduction.* 5th ed. Belmont, CA: Wadsworth, Cengage Learning.

Sherry, J., S. Mookherji, and L. Ryan. 2009. *The five-year evaluation of the Global Fund to fight AIDS, TB and malaria: Synthesis of study areas 1, 2 and 3.* Calverton, MD: Macro International, Inc.

Simon, J., K. Yeboah-Antwi, A. Schapira, M. K. Cham, R. Barber-Madden, and M. I. Brooks. 2011. *External evaluation of the president's malaria initiative: Final report executive summary.* Washington, DC: The Global Health Technical Assistance Project.

Stern, E., N. Stame, J. Mayne, K. Forss, R. Davies, and B. Befani. 2012. *Broadening the range of designs and methods for impact evaluations: Report of a study commissioned by the Department for International Development. (working paper 38).* United Kingdom: Department for International Development.

Tougher, S., Y. Ye, J. H. Amuasi, I. A. Kourgueni, R. Thomson, C. Goodman, A. G. Mann, R. Ren, B. A. Willey, C. A. Adegoke, A. Amin, D. Ansong, K. Bruxvoort, D. A. Diallo, G. Diap, C. Festo, B. Johanes, E. Juma, A. Kalolella, O. Malam, B. Mberu, S. Ndiaye, S. B. Nguah, M. Seydou, M. Taylor, S. T. Rueda, M. Wamukoya, F. Arnold, and K. Hanson. 2012. Effect of the affordable medicines facility—malaria (AMFm) on the availability, price, and market share of quality-assured artemisinin-based combination therapies in seven countries: A before-and-after analysis of outlet survey data. *Lancet* 380(9857):1916–1926.

Verguet, S., R. Laxminarayan, and D. T. Jamison. 2014. Universal public finance of tuberculosis treatment in india: An extended cost-effectiveness analysis. *Health Economics.*

Vickerman, P., C. Watts, S. Delany, M. Alary, H. Rees, and L. Heise. 2006. The importance of context: Model projections on how microbicide impact could be affected by the underlying epidemiologic and behavioral situation in 2 African settings. *Sexually Transmitted Diseases* 33(6):397–405.

White, H., and D. Phillips. 2012. *Addressing attribution of cause and effect in small n impact evaluations: Towards an integrated framework (working paper 15).* New Delhi, India: International Initiative for Impact Evaluation (3ie).

WHO (World Health Organization). 2000. *The world health report 2000. Health systems: Improving performance.* Geneva, Switzerland: World Health Organization.

Appendix A

Statement of Task

An ad hoc committee will plan and conduct a 2-day public workshop on "Lessons Learned in the Conduct of Large-Scale, Complex, Multi-National Global Health Program Evaluations." The scope of the workshop will encompass key points learned in the execution of the IOM's second evaluation of PEPFAR (to be released in February 2013), the 2009 evaluation of the Global Fund, the 2011 evaluation of the President's Malaria Initiative (PMI), the 2012 evaluation of the Affordable Medicines Facility–malaria (AMFm), and 1–2 examples of non-health development assistance programs. The workshop will focus on transferable insights gained across the spectrum of choosing the evaluator, framing the evaluation, developing the methodological approach, implementing the study plan, gathering, assessing and analyzing the data, synthesizing the findings and recommendations, and communicating the key messages. The workshop will illuminate the relative benefits and limitations of quantitative, qualitative, and mixed methodologies used for these complex and expensive evaluations.

The workshop will be planned by an appointed, international planning committee and take place in Washington, DC; London, UK; Geneva, Switzerland; or South Africa. The participants will include individuals involved with the execution of the previously mentioned evaluations, representatives of the agencies that commissioned the evaluations, experts in a range of evaluation methods, and diverse users of the published evaluations. The discussions will reflect the reality of executing these kinds of evaluations, rather than evaluation theory. The goal is to extend evaluation methodologies by capturing lessons learned. Representatives of foundations, bilateral and multilateral governmental donors, and NGOs also will be invited to attend and participate as will representatives of the academic, international organization, and scientific communities involved with the execution of evaluations of this type.

The format of the workshop will include presentations, moderated panel discussions, and small group consultations for participants to explore the application of lessons learned to future work. The workshop may be webcast and archived if resources allow and a rapporteur-authored book length report will summarize the proceedings and be published for a global audience by the U.S. National Academies Press.

Specific issues to be explored in the workshop include

1. Perspectives on terminology, levels of evidence, and the nature of evidence.
2. Issues in program evaluation design, including determination of appropriate evaluation questions to be addressed with appropriately matched methods; prospective and retrospective approaches; longitudinal versus cross-sectional versus comparison approaches; and purposeful sampling to maximize feasibility and representativeness.
3. Methodological issues in evaluating complex and dynamic programs while they are evolving.
4. Data sources, data quality assurance, and post-evaluation data access issues.
5. The complementary utility of quantitative and qualitative mixed methods approaches to evaluation; creating an effective interdisciplinary scientific team.
6. Managing the challenge of program contribution versus attribution.
7. Component analysis.
8. Framing and communicating key findings and recommendations in terms that are useful to stakeholders.
9. Using evaluations to guide future program implementation and program improvement.
10. Using evaluations to guide or influence policy and funding decisions.

Appendix B

Workshop Agenda

Workshop on Evaluation Methods for Large-Scale,
Complex, Multi-National Global Health Initiatives
January 7–8, 2014
Wellcome Trust, Gibbs Building, 215 Euston Road, London

GOALS OF THE WORKSHOP

The goal of the workshop was to elucidate the decision making needed and options available to develop and implement a credible, rigorous evaluation that is also feasible, affordable, and maximally matched to the priority evaluation questions, aims, and audiences. Workshop sessions identified the resultant gains and trade-offs from different choices across the key elements that make up a large-scale evaluation.

The workshop convened relevant stakeholders, including evaluators and users of large-scale evaluations as well as others interested in evaluation methods, to present and discuss insights gained and transferrable lessons learned from the conduct of recent evaluations of the U.S. President's Emergency Plan for AIDS Relief; the Global Fund to Fight AIDS, Tuberculosis, and Malaria; the U.S. President's Malaria Initiative; the Affordable Medicines Facility–malaria; and other large-scale global initiatives.

For the core examples chosen, *large-scale* refers to initiatives with a total cumulative budget over multiple years in at least the hundreds of millions of U.S. dollars. *Multi-national* means implementation on a global scale, including multiple countries and regions or subregions of the world. *Complexity* refers to several dimensions of the initiative. One is that the initiative encompasses multiple different components, such as varied types of interventions and programs implemented in varied settings; systems-strengthening efforts; capacity building; efforts to influence policy change; and utilization of heath diplomacy to achieve the aims of initiative. Another dimension of complexity is implementation at varied levels within partner countries through a large number of diverse, multi-sectoral partners, including an emphasis on local governments and nongovernmental institutions.

While the core examples discussed reflected complex initiatives on this global scale, the intent of the workshop was to also elucidate how the same considerations and decision making can be applied to enhance the credibility, rigor, feasibility, and utility for evaluations that may be on a smaller scale yet share similar features of complexity.

This workshop was sponsored by the Bill & Melinda Gates Foundation, the Doris Duke Charitable Foundation, the Wellcome Trust, and the William and Flora Hewlett Foundation.

AGENDA

Tuesday, January 7, 2014

8:00A – 8:30A   **Registration and Breakfast**

8:30A – 8:45A   **Welcoming Remarks and Overview of Workshop Agenda**
> Ann Kurth, New York University, *Planning Committee Chair*

8:45A – 9:15A   **Setting the Stage: Workshop Framing and Cross-cutting Issues**
> Simon Hearn, Overseas Development Institute/BetterEvaluation Initiative

9:15A – 10:45A   **Panel 1: Framing the evaluation, choosing the evaluator, and establishing the governance structure for the evaluation**

OBJECTIVES OF THE PANEL:
At the end of this session, workshop participants will be able to identify and understand the key considerations and decisions needed to:

- Identify the evaluation goals, develop and prioritize the evaluation questions, and define the audience and the intended uses.
- Understand how decisions and trade-offs in

choosing the type of evaluator and in setting up
the governance structure for the evaluation may
be affected by the different aims/audiences and the
degree to which they are aligned.
- Understand how the options and trade-offs in
  choosing the type of evaluator and in setting up the
  governance structure contribute to designing and
  conducting the best evaluation for the available
  funds.
- Identify how to understand, ensure, and assess the
  value and utility of the evaluation and its findings.

PANELISTS:
Overview Speaker/Moderator: Jon Simon, Boston
University, *Planning Committee Member*

Discussants: Chris Whitty, UK Department for
               International Development
               Ryuichi Komatsu, Global Fund to Fight
                   AIDS, Tuberculosis, and Malaria
               Deborah Rugg, United Nations
                   Inspection and Evaluation Division
               Carmela Green-Abate, Country
                   Coordinator, PEPFAR Ethiopia
               Robert Black, Johns Hopkins University

10:45A – 11:15A BREAK

11:15A – 1:00P   **Panel 2: Developing the evaluation design and
                 methodological approaches**

                 OBJECTIVES OF THE PANEL:
                 At the end of this session, workshop participants will
                 understand the following:

                 - The importance of mixed methods approaches to
                   evaluate complex initiatives and to understand not
                   only whether an effect was achieved but also how
                   and why.

- The importance of strategically thinking through different options for methods and how they can be matched to the evaluation aims/questions, the available data, and the feasibility of implementing the methods with appropriate rigor (design that is "fit for purpose" and feasible).
- How to recognize, understand, and grapple with the complexity of the initiative being evaluated and the context in which that initiative is implemented—this affects, for example, attribution versus contribution designs and expectations for findings.
- The importance of planning for and building flexibility into the design.

PANELISTS:
Moderator: Kara Hanson, London School of Hygiene and Tropical Medicine, *Planning Committee Member*

Presentation: Evaluation of PEPFAR
   Deborah Rugg, United Nations Inspection and Evaluation Division

Presentation: Evaluation of Global Fund
   Daniel Low-Beer, Global Fund to Fight AIDS, Tuberculosis, and Malaria

Presentation: Evaluation of the Affordable Medicines Facility–malaria
   Catherine Goodman, London School of Hygiene and Tropical Medicine

Presentation: Illustration of Good Practices for Complex Evaluation Design
   Elliot Stern, Lancaster University

1:00P – 2:15P   LUNCH

2:15P – 4:00P   **Panel 3: Mapping data sources and gathering and assessing the data**

OBJECTIVES OF THE PANEL:
At the end of this session, workshop participants will understand the following:

- The importance of and strategies for identifying and assessing potential data sources and mapping these to the evaluation questions and the methodological approaches being considered (data that is "fit for purpose").
- The key elements of assessing data sources:
  - Availability
  - Accessibility (including data ownership issues and data sharing agreements)
  - Quality
  - Feasibility of gathering/accessing the identified data

PANELISTS:
Overview Speaker/Moderator: Ann Kurth, New York University, *Planning Committee Chair*

Discussants: Martin Vaessen, ICF, *Planning Committee Member*
Kara Hanson, London School of Hygiene and Tropical Medicine, *Planning Committee Member*
Jon Simon, Boston University, *Planning Committee Member*
Batya Elul, Columbia University
Victoria Fan, Center for Global Development
Peter Elias, University of Warwick

4:00P – 4:30P   BREAK

4:30P – 6:00P   **Panel 4: Analyzing data using triangulation in a mixed methods evaluation to reach overall findings, conclusions, and recommendations**

OBJECTIVES OF THE PANEL:
At the end of this session, workshop participants will understand the following key considerations in data analysis and interpretation for a complex, mixed methods evaluation:

- Data analysis and interpretation within each data type/method according to the methodological standards of rigor for that method (i.e., avoiding "mixed-up" methods).
- Triangulation among the findings from mixed methods to achieve an overall, integrated analysis and interpretation to arrive at major conclusions and recommendations.
- Triangulation among investigators.
  - Among members of the evaluation team
  - Use of expert/advisory panels
  - Use of internal or external reviewers

PANELISTS:
Overview Speaker/Moderator: Carlo Carugi, Global Environment Facility

Discussants: Jon Simon, Boston University, *Planning Committee Member*
Catherine Goodman, London School of Hygiene and Tropical Medicine
Sangeeta Mookherji, George Washington University
Bridget Kelly, Institute of Medicine

6:00P – 6:15P   **Day 1 Wrap-Up**
Ann Kurth, New York University, *Planning Committee Chair*

Wednesday, January 8, 2014

8:00A – 8:30A   **Registration and Breakfast**

8:30A – 8:45A   **Welcoming Remarks: Brief Reflection on Day 1 and Overview of Day 2 Agenda**
Ann Kurth, New York University, *Planning Committee Chair*

8:45A – 10:15A   **Panel 5: Using the evaluation findings and communicating the key messages**

OBJECTIVES OF THE PANEL:
At the end of this session, workshop participants will understand the following:

- Complexity of diverse uses and audiences for large-scale evaluations (e.g., accountability to funders/legislators; program improvement at headquarter, implementer, and country program levels; advocacy to continue initiative; public awareness).
- Importance of matching the message, the messenger, and the audience (communication that is "fit for purpose").
- Challenges with tracking the use of large-scale evaluation findings.

PANELISTS:
Moderator: Sir George Alleyne, University of West Indies, *Planning Committee Member*

Discussants: Bernard Nahlen, President's Malaria Initiative
Dorothy Muroki, FHI360, *Planning Committee Member*
Ian Goldman, Department of Performance Monitoring and Evaluation, Government of South Africa
Kimberly Scott, Institute of Medicine

10:15A – 10:45A   BREAK

10:45A – 12:15P   **Concurrent Sessions—Block 1**

1A: Lessons from Large-Scale Program Evaluation on a Not-Quite-as-Large Scale

Moderator: Dorothy Muroki, FHI360, *Planning Committee Member*

Presenters: Margaret Kruk, Columbia University
Padma Chandrasekaran, The Chennai Angels
Tanya Marchant, London School of Hygiene and Tropical Medicine

1B: Evolving Methods in Evaluation Science

Moderator: Sir George Alleyne, University of West Indies, *Planning Committee Member*

Presenters: Geoff Wong, Queen Mary University of London
Emmanuela Gakidou, Institute for Health Metrics and Evaluation
Caine Rolleston, University of London

1C: Strategic Evaluation Design Troubleshooting: "Bring Your Own" Evaluation Challenge
Workshop participants are invited to bring their own current evaluation design challenges for a roundtable discussion of design options and solutions with evaluation expert panelists and colleagues.

Facilitator: Kimberly Scott, Institute of Medicine

Evaluation experts: Tessie Catsambas, EnCompass LLC
Sharon Knight, East Carolina University

12:15P – 1:30P   **LUNCH: Workshop Feedback Session**
Facilitator: Sharon Knight, East Carolina University

1:30P – 3:00P   **Concurrent Sessions—Block 2**

2A: Applying Qualitative Methods to Evaluation on a Large Scale

Moderator: Kate Meck, Institute of Medicine

Presenters: Sharon Knight, East Carolina University
Tessie Catsambas, EnCompass LLC

2B: Applying Quantitative Methods for Evaluation on a Large Scale

Moderator: Martin Vaessen, ICF International

Presenters: Eran Bendavid, Stanford University
Charlotte Watts, London School of Hygiene and Tropical Medicine
Rachel Nugent, University of Washington

2C: Strategic Evaluation Design Troubleshooting: "Bring Your Own" Evaluation Challenge
Workshop participants are invited to bring their own current evaluation design challenges for a roundtable discussion of design options and solutions with evaluation expert panelists and colleagues.

Facilitator: Bridget Kelly, Institute of Medicine

Evaluation experts: Batya Elul, Columbia University
Sangeeta Mookherji, George Washington University
Joanna Schellenberg, London School of Hygiene and Tropical Medicine

3:00P – 3:30P   BREAK

3:30P – 4:45P   **Panel 6: Envisioning a future evaluation**

OBJECTIVE OF THE PANEL:
Synthesize key messages of the workshop by applying them in a hypothetical design exercise.

PANELISTS:
Moderator: Elliot Stern, Lancaster University

Presenters: Sanjeev Sridharan, Evaluation Centre for Complex Health Interventions, University of Toronto/St. Michaels's Hospital
Charlotte Watts, London School of Hygiene and Tropical Medicine

4:45P – 5:15P   **Summary Highlights of the Workshop and Reflections on Key Outcomes**
Ruth Levine, William and Flora Hewlett Foundation

Additional Reflections
Mary Bassett, Doris Duke Charitable Foundation
Gina Dallabetta, Bill & Melinda Gates Foundation
Jimmy Whitworth, Wellcome Trust

5:15P – 5:30P   **Closing Remarks and Adjournment**
Ann Kurth, New York University, *Planning Committee Chair*

Appendix C

Participant Biographies

Sir George Alleyne, a native of Barbados, became Director of the Pan American Health Organization (PAHO), Regional Office of WHO on February 1, 1995, and completed a second 4-year term on January 31, 2003. In 2003 he was elected Director Emeritus of PAHO. From February 2003 until December 2010 he was the UN Secretary General's Special Envoy for HIV/AIDS in the Caribbean. In October 2003 he was appointed Chancellor of the University of the West Indies. He currently holds an Adjunct Professorship at the Bloomberg School of Public Health, Johns Hopkins University. Sir Alleyne has received numerous awards in recognition of his work, including prestigious decorations and national honors from many countries of the Americas. In 1990, he was made Knight Bachelor by Her Majesty Queen Elizabeth II for his services to Medicine. In 2001, he was awarded the Order of the Caribbean Community, the highest honor that can be conferred on a Caribbean national.

Mary T. Bassett is a Program Director at the Doris Duke Charitable Foundation, leading its African Health Initiative, an effort that focuses on strengthening health systems in projects under way in Ghana, Mozambique, Rwanda, Tanzania, and Zambia. In late 2011, she additionally assumed leadership for the Child Abuse Prevention Program, which for 10 years has made grants aimed at preventing child maltreatment.

Eran Bendavid is an infectious diseases physician, an Assistant Professor of Medicine at Stanford University, and an affiliate at the Center for

129

Health Policy and the Woods Institute for the Environment. He studies how economic, political, and natural environments affect population health in developing countries using a mix of experimental, epidemiologic, econometric, qualitative, modeling, and demographic tools. Bendavid blends methodological innovation and practical experience working with local and international organizations, including the Clinton Health Access Initiative (Liberia), the Desmond Tutu HIV Foundation (South Africa), and the Kenya Medical Research Institute, to produce insights and strategies for health improvements. He led empirical evaluations of international malaria and HIV control initiatives. His studies on the relationship between PEPFAR and population health outcomes have appeared in the *Journal of the American Medical Association* and the *Annals of Internal Medicine*.

Robert E. Black is the Professor and Director of the Institute for International Programs in the Department of International Health, Johns Hopkins Bloomberg School of Public Health in Baltimore, Maryland. Black is trained in medicine, infectious diseases, and epidemiology. He served as an epidemiologist at CDC and at institutions in Bangladesh and Peru on research related to childhood infectious diseases and nutrition. His current research includes field trials of vaccines, micronutrients and other nutritional interventions, effectiveness studies of health programs, and evaluation of preventive and curative health services in low- and middle-income countries. His other interests are the use of evidence in guiding policy and programs, including estimates of burden of disease, and the strengthening of public health training. He has more than 500 scientific journal publications and is co-editor of the textbook *Global Health*.

Carlo Carugi leads the country-level evaluation stream of work at the GEF Independent Evaluation Office since July 2009. One of his main responsibilities in this position is to lead the design, strengthening, updating, and refinement of evaluation methods, tools, and processes in use, aiming at fostering the analytical rigor as well as the independence, credibility, and utility of the GEF country-level evaluations. Triangulation analysis in mixed methods evaluations has been one of Carugi's main interests since he joined the GEF Independent Evaluation Office. Another major area of interest is the evaluation process. In his work Carugi endeavors to foster inclusiveness and learning with evaluation users and stakeholders and in particular with national partners by promoting a much stronger role for countries in the evaluation of development policies, programs, and projects, without compromising the independence and rigor of evaluations. Carugi has 25 years of experience in environment and development, 15 of which were spent in developing countries. He has been involved in designing, managing, and directly conducting evaluations since 1991. All along his professional career he conducted a number of project, program, strategic, thematic, and country-level evaluations for the European Commission, Italy, Food and Agriculture Association (FAO), and others. Carugi holds an M.Sc. in Agricultural Science and an M.Sc. in Environment and Development.

Anastasia (Tessie) Tzavaras Catsambas is President of EnCompass LLC and brings 30 years of experience in evaluation and management of international programs. Catsambas is an innovator and practitioner in appreciative evaluation methods. She brings rich field experience to her annual trainings at the American Evaluation Association's Annual Conference since 2002 on qualitative methods, including: Appreciative Inquiry for Evaluation; Improvement and Learning Collaboratives; Evaluation Capacity Development; and Advocacy for Evaluation. She has co-authored two chapters on appreciative evaluation (Preskill & Coghlan, *New Directions for Evaluation* #100, 2003), and co-authored with Hallie Preskill a book titled *Reframing Evaluation Through Appreciative Inquiry* (Sage Publications, 2006). Catsambas' recent work included an evaluation of the USAID Policy, Planning and Learning Bureau (PPL); a 2-year evaluation of the Gates-funded Centre for Tobacco Control in Africa (CTCA) housed in Makerere University in Uganda, and implemented by WHO; and a 2-year evaluation of the Gates-funded Ministerial Leadership Initiative (MLI) implemented by The Aspen Institute. Catsambas holds a bachelor's degree in economics and political science from the College of Wooster and a master's degree in public policy from Harvard University. She has trained with the late Dr. W. Edwards Deming in Quality Management. She is fluent in French and Greek, and speaks Spanish. Since 2012, Catsambas has served on the Board of the International Organization for Cooperation in Evaluation as Secretary, on the Executive Group of EvalPartners, and Co-Chair of the Enabling Environment Task Force. Catsambas is committed to building equity-focused and gender-responsive evaluation globally.

Padma Chandrasekaran has had 10 plus years experience in the nonprofit health and human development sector with the Bill & Melinda Gates Foundation and more than 18 years in for-profit information technology and venture investing. Chandrasekaran's areas of professional expertise and interest include strategy, program management and evaluation, and analytics and the use of data for decision making. Between 2003 and 2011, she worked full time for the Bill & Melinda Gates Foundation. She initially held responsibilities for strategy development, program management, and impact evaluation for HIV, maternal, and child health programming. She was also responsible subsequently for the foundation's initiatives in vaccine development and delivery in India. Chandrasekaran designed, developed, and implemented strategy and systems for routine monitoring and management, as well as long-term impact and economic evaluation for Avahan, a key population-focused HIV prevention program covering some 220,000 sex workers, 80,000 high-risk men who have sex with men, and 20,000 intravenous drug users in six states. She also developed the initial program and program evaluation design for the foundation's maternal and child health programming in Bihar. Chandrasekaran continues to consult for the foundation's global activities in specific areas related to routine data systems and health economics. Prior to the foundation, her private-sector experience (1984–2003) followed a standard gradient of software developer, manager, executive officer, and entrepreneur in the Information Technology sector in India, the United States, and the United Kingdom. She was a co-founder of Sify Ltd., India's first Internet company and part of the team that took it public on Nasdaq in 1999. She subsequently founded, ran, and sold a Web services software technology company. She is currently an active angel investor in startups in health/life sciences, big data analytics, IT, and education. She is an Executive Committee of The Chennai Angels, an angel investment group, and a Charter Member of The Indus Entrepreneurs, a global nonprofit dedicated to furthering the cause of entrepreneurship. She is also on the board of directors of several companies in India. Chandrasekaran holds a bachelor's degree in mathematics and statistics from the University of Calcutta; an M.B.A. from the Indian Institute of Management, Ahmedabad, and a master's degree in telecommunications from the University of San Francisco, California. She has been lead or co-author for peer-reviewed publications published in journals including the *Lancet ID*, *J-Aids*, and *BMJ-STI*.

Gina Dallabetta is a Senior Program Officer at the Bill & Melinda Gates Foundation. Dallabetta joined the Foundation's Avahan-India AIDS Initiative in January 2005. She has 20 years of experience in HIV programming. Previously, Dallabetta was Director of the Prevention Department of the HIV/AIDS Institute of Family Health International (FHI). The department was responsible for sexually transmitted infection, behavior change communication, monitoring and evaluation, and related operations research in more than 40 countries in Africa, Asia, the Caribbean, Eastern Europe, Latin America, and the Middle East. She co-edited *Control of Sexually Transmitted Diseases: A Handbook for the Design and Management of Programs*, the first book ever produced for managers of Sexually Transmitted Infection programs in developing countries, now considered a standard supplementary text for graduate programs in international health.

Peter Elias is a labor economist. He has degrees in chemistry from the University of Manchester (1967) and business administration from the University of Sheffield (1970). He worked in industry and government before commencing his doctoral studies in labor economics and econometrics at the University of California, Berkeley (1971–1975). On completion of his doctorate he joined the Institute for Employment Research at the University of Warwick in 1975 and has been continuously employed there since that date. His research interests range from the evaluation of large-scale government programs designed to affect labor market behavior, statistical monitoring of the status of particular groups in the labor market, the study of occupational change, and the relationship between further and higher education, vocational training, and labor market outcomes. He has developed methods for the measurement and analysis of labor market dynamics and has a keen interest in the classification of labor market activities. On October 1, 2004, he was appointed as the ESRC Strategic Advisor for Data Resources, a post that he will hold until 2016. In his capacity as an advisor to the Economic and Social Research Council he has had responsibility for the development, implementation, maintenance, and revision of the *National Strategy for Data Resources for the Social Sciences*. He has helped launch *Understanding Society*, the UK Household Longitudinal Study, new data services to provide access to administrative data, and a secure data environment for access to sensitive data. He also worked to secure funding for the new Birth Cohort Study (Life Study). In 2011 he was awarded a CBE for services to the social sciences. In December 2013 he accepted an honorary professorship at the Institute of Child Health, University College London, and was appointed as the Deputy Director of the Life Study.

Batya Elul is Assistant Professor of Clinical Epidemiology at Columbia University's Mailman School of Public Health and Director of Strategic Information at ICAP, a large center at Columbia University that focuses on implementation support, capacity building, and technical assistance for HIV and related health programs in resource-limited settings. In her role at ICAP, she oversees a team of 15 professionals in New York and more than 50 in sub-Saharan Africa and Central Asia to conduct monitoring, evaluation, and surveillance activities for more than 30 grants related to HIV service scale-up totaling $135 million/year. Collectively, the Strategic Information Unit collects, manages, analyzes, and uses innovative approaches to disseminate high-quality data on more than 1.7 million people enrolled in HIV care and more than 750,000 who have initiated antiretroviral therapy. She also leads efforts to provide technical assistance to and build capacity of Ministries of Health to plan and implement monitoring and evaluation, surveillance, and research activities that generate relevant and timely data for evidence-based decision making.

Victoria Fan is a research fellow and health economist at the Center for Global Development. Her research focuses on the design and evaluation of health policies and programs as well as of global health donors and agencies and their policies. Fan joined the center after completing her doctorate at Harvard School of Public Health where she wrote her dissertation on health systems in India. Fan has worked at various nongovernmental organizations in Asia (BRAC, Self Employed Women's Association, and Tzu Chi), and different units at Harvard University (Initiative for Global Health, Global Equity Initiative, Program in Health Financing) and has served as a consultant for the World Bank and WHO. Fan's ongoing research interests include health insurance and conditional cash transfers in Asia as well as health aid in Afghanistan and Haiti. Fan's most recent publication is a report on *More Health for the Money*, which can be accessed at morehealthforthemoney. org.

Emmanuela Gakidou is Professor of Global Health and Director of Education and Training at the Institute for Health Metrics and Evaluation (IHME) at the University of Washington. She also leads the institute's research activities in the area of evaluations. In addition, she is currently a Faculty Affiliate for the Center for Statistics and the Social Sciences at the University of Washington. Her research interests are impact evaluation and methods development for analytical challenges in global health. Examples of current research projects include the evaluation of Avahan—a large HIV prevention program in India, the development of a time series of educational attainment for all countries from 1960 to present, the measurement of adult mortality in developing countries, and the measurement of economic status through health surveys. Before joining IHME, Gakidou was a research associate at the Harvard Initiative for Global Health and the Institute for Quantitative Social Science. Prior to moving to Harvard University, Gakidou worked as a health economist at WHO, where she led work on the measurement of health inequalities. Apart from being instrumental in the founding of IHME, Gakidou is passionate about training the next generation of leaders in the field of health metrics and evaluation. She created and is directing the two fellowship programs at IHME, and is coordinating the overall curriculum and degree programs the institute offers through the Department of Global Health. Originally from Greece, Gakidou moved to the United States for higher education and received her degrees—a bachelor of arts, a master of international health economics, and a Ph.D. in health policy—from Harvard University.

Ian Goldman is Head of Evaluation and Research in the Department of Performance M&E (monitoring and evaluation) in the South African Presidency. Ian has worked in rural development, decentralization, local economic development, and community-driven development in 18 countries, working with NGOs and local, provincial, or national governments. His passion is in action learning approaches for development, and the South African system is learning centered. The policy underlying the system was approved in November 2011, and 38 evaluations have been completed, are under way, or about to start, representing several billion pounds of government spending.

Catherine Goodman is a senior lecturer in health economics and policy in the Department of Global Health and Development at the London School of Hygiene and Tropical Medicine. She has 15 years of experience in applied health systems research in low- and middle-income settings, with a focus on private-sector provision, health care financing and governance, and the economics of malaria control. Goodman has extensive experience in the economic evaluation of malaria control strategies. She has participated in numerous projects on access to antimalarial treatment. This has included the Independent Evaluation of AMFm, a multi-national antimalarial subsidy program; health facility assessments of the introduction of malaria rapid diagnostic tests; and analysis of antimalarial distribution chains under ACTwatch. She has a strong interest in methods for studying private-sector provision in general.

Carmela Green-Abate is a pediatrician with more than 35 years of experience in international health, with a special focus on child health. She has been PEPFAR Coordinator in Ethiopia since January 2009 but has lived in Ethiopia for 40 years. Previously she worked for Catholic Relief Services, latterly on their PEPFAR multicountry HIV and AIDS treatment program—AIDSRelief, where she was the Deputy Chief of Party for Africa. In that position she travelled extensively throughout Africa. She worked for USAID in Ethiopia from 1991 to 1997, initially on their orphans and vulnerable children's program and subsequently as Senior Technical Advisor for Health. She was involved in the design of the first U.S. government–supported HIV/AIDS program in Ethiopia and then in the design and oversight of their first health-sector program. Prior to that, she worked in the Department of Pediatrics in Addis Ababa University for 14 years, in charge of neonatal services and undergraduate programs. She has been actively involved in the Ethiopian NGO sector, most notably as the founder of the Gemini Foundation, which assists very disadvantaged families with twins living in the slums of Addis Ababa. The Gemini Foundation pioneered youth involvement in creative arts as a tool for development. As part of this initiative, GemTV, winner of the 2012 One World Media Special Award, was the first community video production company in Ethiopia, spearheading docu-drama films for behavior change. The international recognized Adugna Dance Company is the only contemporary dance company in Ethiopia, with its dancers performing in many prestigious venues in London and New York. Adugna also works at the community level with marginalized groups as well as with young people with disabilities.

Kara Hanson is Professor of Health System Economics at the London School of Hygiene and Tropical Medicine and head of the Department of Global Health and Development. She holds degrees from McGill University, Montreal, Canada; University of Cambridge, UK; and Harvard University. She has nearly 25 years of experience researching health systems in low- and middle-income countries, providing policy advice and input, and teaching health economics and supervising Ph.D. projects. Her research focuses on the financing and organization of health services, and has included research on scaling up health services, the impact of community-based health insurance, equity consequences of user fees and their removal, and expanding domestic fiscal space. She has worked extensively on the role of the private sector in health systems, identifying the opportunities and limitations of the private sector in improving the efficiency, quality, and responsiveness of health systems. Her work in this area includes studying the demand for private health services in Sri Lanka and Cyprus, developing innovative methods for studying private-sector supply chains for antimalarial medicines, and evaluating a voucher scheme for delivering insecticide-treated mosquito nets. She was a co-investigator for the Independent Evaluation of AMFm for the Global Fund. She is co-Research Director of RESYST—Resilient and Responsive Health Systems, which is a UK-DFID funded research consortium bringing together researchers from India, Kenya, Nigeria, South Africa, Tanzania, Thailand, Vietnam, and the United Kingdom. The RESYST program includes research on health financing, health workers, and governance and leadership in the health sector, together with a focus on capacity development and encouraging the uptake of research findings into policy and practice. She has published widely in health economics and public health journals, and was editor of *Health Policy and Planning* from 2001 to 2008.

Simon Hearn has spent 10 years working in international development, first for a small research firm, and for the past 6 years at the Overseas Development Institute where he is currently a Research Fellow. He specializes in understanding the interface between research and policy, particularly the role that evaluation and organizational learning can play in improving programs and systems. He is the global coordinator for the Outcome Mapping Learning Community, a global group of trainers, specialists, and users of outcome mapping, and a founding member and community facilitator of BetterEvaluation, an international initiative to improve evaluation capacity. He is an experienced trainer and facilitator and has advised a number of international development programs on measuring and evaluation, policy-influencing strategies, and network management.

Sharon Knight is a Professor of Health Education in the College of Health and Human Performance at East Carolina University, Greenville, North Carolina. Her area of research interest and expertise is qualitative research. She most recently served as the qualitative consultant on an IOM global, mixed methods evaluation of the PEPFAR program. Her 25 years as a qualitative researcher and health educator in higher education was preceded by a 12-year nursing career that included service in the U.S. Army Nurse Corps.

Ryuichi Komatsu is currently Senior Advisor, TERG, at the Global Fund Secretariat. He facilitates coordination within and outside the Global Fund Secretariat to implement the work plan of the TERG and advises on policy making and strategic options and decisions of the Global Fund management. He is responsible for providing support to the TERG in the implementation of the TERG work plan including the management of independent evaluations. His experience at the Global Fund since 2005 includes managing teams on strategic information and impact evaluation. Previously, he worked for the National Institute of Population and Social Security Research in Japan and the East-West Center in the United States as well as various governmental and NGOs in different countries as part of assignments.

Margaret E. Kruk is an Assistant Professor in Health Policy and Management at Columbia University Mailman School of Public Health. Previously, she was Policy Advisor for Health at the Millennium Project, an advisory body to the UN Secretary-General on the Millennium Development Goals, and a manager in the health care practice at McKinsey and Company in New York. Kruk holds an M.D. from McMaster University and an M.P.H. (Health Policy and Management) from Harvard University. On completing her family medicine residency, she practiced family and emergency medicine in remote northern Ontario, Canada. She conducts quantitative health systems research in low-income countries, particularly in sub-Saharan Africa, with funding from NIH, CDC, USAID, and private foundations. She studies health care utilization, population preferences for care, and the performance of health systems in improving health, equity, and financial protection. Kruk uses novel methods to evaluate large-scale health programs and is interested in improving research design and measurement in implementation science. She has been a consultant to governments, WHO, United Nations Population Fund, and the World Bank, and she has published more than 50 research papers.

Ann Kurth is Professor of Nursing, Medicine, and Public Health at New York University (NYU) and Associate Dean for Research at the NYU Global Institute of Public Health. As a clinically trained epidemiologist Kurth's research focuses on sexual and reproductive health as well as on global health system strengthening and using information and communication technologies among other approaches. Her work has been funded by NIH, the Bill & Melinda Gates Foundation, UNAIDS, CDC, and others, for studies conducted in the United States and internationally. She has published more than 110 peer-reviewed articles, book chapters, and scholarly monographs, including one of the first books on women and HIV. Kurth received a Ph.D. in epidemiology from the University of Washington, an M.S.N. in nurse-midwifery from Yale University, and an M.P.H. in population and family health from Columbia University. Kurth was a member of the IOM/National Academy of Science Committee on PEPFAR2 Evaluation. Kurth is an elected member of the IOM, a Fellow of the American Academy of Nursing and of the New York Academy of Medicine, and a member of the 2014–2018 U.S. Preventive Services Task Force.

Ruth Levine is a development economist and expert in international development, global health, and education, and she serves as the director of the Foundation's Global Development and Population Program. Before joining the foundation, Levine was a deputy assistant administrator in the Bureau of Policy, Planning, and Learning at USAID. In that role, she led the development of the agency's evaluation policy. Previously, she spent nearly a decade at the Center for Global Development, an international policy research institute in Washington, DC. There, she served as a Senior Fellow and vice president for programs and operations. Levine is the author of scores of books and professional publications, including a recent pair of influential reports from the Center for Global Development on development and adolescent girls: *Girls Count: A Global Investment & Action Agenda* and *Start with a Girl: A New Agenda for Global Health*. She also is co-author of the highly regarded report *When Will We Ever Learn?: Improving Lives through Impact Evaluation*. Levine holds a B.S. in biochemistry from Cornell University and a Ph.D. in economic demography from the Johns Hopkins University.

Daniel Low-Beer is Head of Impact, Results, and Evaluation at the Global Fund. He has 20 years' experience in global health, directing programs at global and country level, working with government, NGOs, and the private sector. He worked with WHO in the early 1990s, collaborating with Ministries of Health in Africa and Asia and leading the first Global Burden of HIV study. He then gained management and strategy experience in the private sector, before directing a unit on Health and Population Evaluation and a master's course at Cambridge University. At the Global Fund he has led the development of results-based financing, counterpart financing, aid effectiveness, and most recently impact evaluation. He has published widely in *Science*, *Nature Medicine*, *Financial Times*, and edited the book *Innovative Health Partnerships: The Diplomacy of Diversity*.

Tanya Marchant is an epidemiologist at the London School of Hygiene and Tropical Medicine. She holds an M.Sc. in medical demography (London School of Hygiene and Tropical Medicine) and a Ph.D. in epidemiology (Swiss Tropical and Public Health Institute). Marchant's research has focused on issues in reproductive, maternal, and newborn health, primarily in sub-Saharan Africa. This began with investigations into fertility preferences and priorities in Gambia and Tanzania and moved onto the prevention of anemia and malaria in pregnancy, including working on the National Evaluation of the Tanzanian National Voucher Scheme. More recently her focus has been on innovations to improve the survival of mothers and newborns in sub-Saharan African and India, and on large-scale measurement of processes, outputs, and outcomes along the continuum of care.

Sangeeta Mookherji is Assistant Professor in the Department of Global Health in the School of Public Health and Health Services at the George Washington University (GWU), Washington, DC. She teaches Global Health Program Evaluation, Case Study Methods for Program Evaluation, and Qualitative and Quantitative Research Methods. She directs the most popular program in the department, Program Design, Monitoring, and Evaluation. Mookherji's research interests include methods for evaluating interventions to improve health systems performance; using case study methods for program and systems evaluation; urban health; tuberculosis control; and maternal and child health. Her current research includes using multiple case studies to understand what drives improvements in routine immunization performance in sub-Saharan Africa; mixed methods evaluation for the Medical Education Partnership Initiative for Africa (MEPI); and using case studies to validate theories of how information systems strengthen health service delivery. Before joining GWU in 2009, Mookherji worked for 15 years evaluating public health programs in Bangladesh, Bhutan, Cambodia, Denmark, India, Morocco, Nigeria, Palestine, Tanzania, Uganda, and the United States, living in five of those countries. She has worked with evaluating a variety of public health program areas, including leading Study Area 2 of the Five-Year Evaluation of the Global Fund; assessing incentives and enablers to improve tuberculosis control systems; metrics for improving urban health systems; as well as financing for immunization, and service quality improvements for reproductive and child health, among others. During that time, she was employed by

Johns Hopkins Bloomberg School of Public Health, Crone and Koch A/S (Denmark), and Management Sciences for Health, and has worked as a consultant for the Asian Development Bank, Danida, USAID, WHO, and the World Bank. She has a B.A. in Comparative Literature and Economics from the University of Pennsylvania and an M.H.S. and Ph.D. from Johns Hopkins. Her Ph.D. dissertation topic was, "Demand for health care among urban slum residents in Dhaka, Bangladesh."

Dorothy Muroki is the Project Director of the USAID-funded Leader-with-Associates *Roads to a Healthy Future (ROADS II)*, multi-year $200 million program. She has 20 years of experience managing health and development programming in sub-Saharan Africa, with core competencies in institutional development and strengthening for nongovernmental, community- and faith-based organizations, participatory training, and monitoring and evaluation. Muroki, a Kenyan national and a communications professional, has extensive experience and demonstrated expertise in mobilizing communities and working with them to contextualize practical and relevant program ideas to address their health challenges. She has successfully directed and managed significant partnerships between communities and local government leadership and key stakeholders, developing sustainability strategies, with a focus on indigenous associations. As the ROADS Project Director, and previously the Deputy ROADS Project Director, she has initiated, led, and been instrumental in developing key program innovations, including the "cluster" community-organizing model and programming to address accessibility and uptake of HIV and health services, gender-based violence, economic strengthening, and food insecurity in the context of HIV and broader health. Muroki has more than 10 years' extensive and direct experience working on regional HIV and health programs that critically and effectively require high-level tact in bilateral relations with country systems, USAID country missions, and transport corridor communities. She has worked on integrating bilateral and community participation through effective feedback loops and plans of action from transport corridor sites to both regional and national policy bodies to inform critical interventions in addressing HIV and health challenges in Burundi, Democratic Republic of Congo, Djibouti, Kenya, Mozambique, Rwanda, South Sudan, Tanzania, Uganda, and Zambia. Muroki holds a bachelor of commerce degree, University of Nairobi, and a master's in communications, Daystar University, Kenya.

Bernard Nahlen has been Deputy Coordinator of the PMI since 2007. He completed his residency in Family Practice at the University of California, San Francisco, before joining CDC in 1986 as an Epidemic Intelligence Service Officer assigned to the Malaria Branch. In 1989, he completed a second residency in Preventive Medicine and later served as Deputy Director of the Los Angeles County AIDS Epidemiology Program. Nahlen's commitment to malaria prevention and control subsequently took him to Kenya in 1992 as Director of the CDC field research station in collaboration with the Kenya Medical Research Institute (KEMRI). In 2000, he served as Senior Technical Advisor to the WHO Malaria Programme. At WHO, he led the Monitoring and Evaluation team as well as the Malaria in Pregnancy team. From 2005 to 2006, Bernard served as a Senior Advisor in the Performance Evaluation and Policy unit of the Global Fund to Fight AIDS, Tuberculosis, and Malaria. He has also authored or co-authored more than 150 articles related to malaria prevention and control.

Rachel Nugent is a development economist with 30 years' experience in policy analysis of agricultural, environmental, and health conditions in developing countries. Since 2000, she has worked on global health policy with particular emphasis on nutrition-related diseases. Nugent was a senior economist at the UN FAO from 1997 to 2000 where she led a multidepart-ment team to study and provide technical support for urban and peri-urban agriculture. In 2000, Nugent joined the Fogarty International Center of NIH. She served as a technical expert to WHO as a member of the inter-national reference group for the Global Strategy on Diet, Physical Activity, and Health. Nugent subsequently was Director of Health and Economic Development at the Population Reference Bureau and Deputy Director of Global Health at the Center for Global Development. In recent years, Nugent has worked on the economic evaluation of health interventions and fiscal policies to address noncommunicable diseases. She was a member of the IOM ad hoc Committee on Cardiovascular Disease in Developing Countries (2009–2010) and chair of the IOM Workshop on Developing a Toolkit for Managing Noncommunicable Diseases (NCDs) in Developing Countries (2011). She is a member of the Lancet NCD Action Group, the NCD Alliance Advisory Team. She is director of the Disease Control Priori-ties Network at the UW Department of Global Health, and editor of the vascular disease volume of that enterprise.

Caine Rolleston graduated from the universities of Oxford and London and has worked on education and international development in a range of countries, including Ethiopia, Ghana, India, Peru, Sri Lanka, and Vietnam. He is currently a lecturer in Education and International Development at the Institute of Education, University of London, teaching on the master's program in Educational Planning, Economics, and International Develop-ment. His research interests focus on issues in the economics of education in developing countries, educational access and equity, privatization, learning metrics and trajectories, and cognitive and noncognitive skills development and measurement. His work draws on longitudinal studies in education and development and employs both quantitative and qualitative research methods. Rolleston has led the education research program at Young Lives, a large-scale international cohort study of childhood poverty based at the University of Oxford since 2011, including designing and implementing school surveys and skills assessments. Previously he worked as a researcher for CREATE (Consortium for Research on Educational Access Transitions and Equity), an international research program based at the University of Sussex. He has conducted a study of low-fee private schooling in Ghana and Nigeria for OSI:PERI (Open Society Initiative: Private Education Research Initiative) and an evaluation the global costs of Education for All (EFA) for the EFA Global Monitoring Report. His doctoral work focused on issues of access to and the economic benefits of education in sub-Saharan Africa, including work on child fosterage and its impact on education, including school drop-outs in migrant labor.

Deborah L. Rugg has more than 30 years of professional international and national evaluation experience and has led international evaluation standards-setting bodies such as the HIV/AIDS Monitoring and Evaluation Reference Group (MERG) where she served as Chair from 2006–2011 and the UN Evaluation Group (UNEG) where she has been serving as Vice Chair since 2012. Since August 2011, Rugg has served as the Director of Inspection and Evaluation Division (IED) in the Office of Inspection and Oversight Services (OIOS), UN Secretariat in New York City. Previously she served as Chief of the Monitoring and Evaluation Division at the Joint UN Programme on AIDS (UNAIDS) in Geneva, Switzerland. Prior to joining UNAIDS in 2005, Rugg was the Associate Director for Monitoring and Evaluation for the Global AIDS Program (GAP) of CDC in Atlanta, Georgia, from 2000 to 2005. While in Atlanta she also served as an Adjunct Associate Professor at Emory University School of Public Health. Prior to that she was Assistant Professor of Health Psychology at the University of California, San Francisco, School of Medicine and then San Diego State University School of Public Health from 1982–1987. She joined CDC in 1987 as an Epidemic Intelligence Service Officer in the Division of HIV/STD Prevention. She has authored or co-authored more than 70 peer-reviewed publications and 30 major agency reports and normative guidances, primarily on evaluation methods in HIV, especially in relation to adolescents, risk groups, and HIV counseling and testing. Rugg currently serves on the IOM Committee to Evaluate the Impact of PEPFAR. She also served on the U.S. National Research Council Panel on Data and Research Priorities for Arresting AIDS in Sub-Saharan Africa. She has a B.A. from the University of Wisconsin in physiological psychology and earned her Ph.D. from the

University of California, San Francisco, School of Medicine in Health Psychology in 1982.

Joanna Schellenberg is a Reader in Epidemiology and International Health based at the London School of Hygiene and Tropical Medicine. After a first degree in mathematics at Oxford she studied for her M.Sc. in biometry at Reading University, and later did a Ph.D. in epidemiology at the University of Basel. She spent almost 10 years living in Tanzania, doing collaborative research work with Ifakara Health Institute. Her main research interest is the development and evaluation of public health interventions for newborn, infant, and child survival in low- and middle-income countries, including evaluation of equity as well as effectiveness. She is principal investigator of IDEAS, a 5-year project funded by the Bill & Melinda Gates Foundation with the aim of improving the evidence base for maternal and newborn health programs in Ethiopia, India, and Nigeria. She also leads a cluster-randomized trial in Tanzania of a behavior-change intervention to improve newborn survival through home-based counseling in pregnancy and the first few days of life; and collaborates on EQUIP, which aims to improve maternal and newborn health in Uganda and Tanzania through quality-improvement approaches linked to information from continuous household surveys.

Jonathon Lee Simon is the Director of the Center for Global Health and Development (CGHD), a multidisciplinary university-wide research center focused on health and socioeconomic development problems among marginalized populations in middle- and low-income settings. Simon is the Robert A. Knox Professor at Boston University (BU). He received his B.S. from the University of California, Berkeley, in Conservation and Resource Studies, and his M.P.H. is from the University of California, Berkeley, School of Public Health. He received his Doctorate of Science from the Harvard School of Public Health, having completed dissertation research on the changing family demography in urban slum communities in Dhaka, Bangladesh. Before joining Boston University, Simon was a Fellow of the Harvard Institute for International Development (HIID). He has been involved with applied child survival research activities for more than 25 years, working in numerous developing countries, most extensively in Africa and South Asia. His primary focus is on policy and program-relevant research related to diarrhea, pneumonia, and malaria with an explicit commitment to strengthening host country child health research capacity as part of all the activities. Simon served in resident positions in Pakistan and Tanzania. He recently served as global team leader of external evaluations of the PMI and the Roll Back Malaria Partnership. He is involved in conducting evaluation research studies of interventions aimed at improving the well-being of orphans and vulnerable children. He is actively engaged with CGHD's Program Evaluation and the Economic Impacts of HIV/AIDS Working Groups. Simon teaches a global public health history course to the incoming M.P.H. students as well as a course on scientific inquiry in the Kilachand Honors College for BU undergraduates in addition to mentoring doctoral students.

Sanjeev Sridharan is Director of the Evaluation Centre for Complex Health Interventions at Li Ka Shing Knowledge Institute at St. Michaels Hospital and Associate Professor at the Department of Health Policy, Management, and Evaluation at the University of Toronto. Prior to his position at Toronto, he was the Head of the Evaluation Program and Senior Research Fellow at the Research Unit in Health, Behaviour and Change at the University of Edinburgh. He is a former Associate Editor of the *American Journal of Evaluation* and is presently on the boards of the *Canadian Journal of Program Evaluation*, the *Journal of Evaluation*, and *Evaluation and Program Planning*.

Elliot Stern is an active member of the international evaluation community. He is a past-President of the European Society, was founding President of the UK Evaluation Society and the IOCE (International Organisation for Cooperation in Evaluation), and edits the journal *Evaluation: The International Journal of Theory, Research and Practice*. He has led major international development evaluation and consultancy projects for DFID, OECD, the European Union, UN agencies, and the World Bank. Stern is Emeritus Professor of Evaluation Research at Lancaster University and is presently Visiting Professor at Bristol University. In recent years he has specialized in evaluation methodology and design and has written extensively on evaluation methods, skills, and practice. In recent years he has developed a particular interest in causal inference and varieties of "impact" evaluation.

Martin Vaessen is a Senior Vice President at ICF International. He is currently in charge of the International Survey Research and Evaluation line of business, concentrating on survey research, with significant emphasis on maternal and child health and nutrition and diseases such as HIV/AIDS and malaria. He came to ICF through the acquisition of Macro International. He joined the renowned DHS project at Macro International in 1985 and was its Project Director for nearly 19 years. Prior to that, he was with the International Statistical Institute from 1973 to 1984 based in London. There he worked as chief of survey operations on the implementation of comparative fertility surveys in 42 countries with the World Fertility Survey. He has worked on survey development and implementation in a large number of developing countries for a variety of donor and implementing agencies. A native of the Netherlands, he has lived and worked in Chile, the United Kingdom, and now in the United States. He has an M.A. in sociology from Tilburg Catholic University in the Netherlands.

Charlotte Watts is Head of the Social and Mathematical Epidemiology Group and founding director of the Gender, Violence and Health Centre, in the Department for Global Health and Development at London School of Health and Tropical Medicine. Originally trained as a mathematician, with further training in epidemiology, economics, and social science methods, she brings a strong multidisciplinary perspective to the complex challenge of addressing HIV and violence against women. She has more than 15 years' experience in international HIV and violence research, including leading randomized controlled trials of violence prevention programs in sub-Saharan Africa, and mathematical modeling projections of the impact and cost-effectiveness of existing and emerging HIV programs in low- and middle-income countries.

Christopher Whitty is Chief Scientific Advisor at the UK's DFID, where he is also director of research and evidence, and currently director of policy. He is seconded from the London School of Hygiene and Tropical Medicine where he is professor of international health. In the DFID he is responsible for the evaluation department and is on the board of the International Initiative on Impact Evaluation (3ie). His research background is in undertaking studies in Africa and Asia, including complex trials and economic and anthropological studies. He trained in medicine (still practices), epidemiology, economics, and law. He is a fellow of the Academy of Medical Sciences, the nearest UK equivalent of the IOM.

Jimmy Whitworth became Head of Population Health at the Wellcome Trust in 2013, having previously been Head of International Activities since 2004. He is responsible for strategy, policy, and developing the scientific portfolio for research on population science and public health research in the United Kingdom and in low- and middle-income countries. Previously he was Professor of International Public Health at the London School of Hygiene and Tropical Medicine. He is a physician, qualifying from Liverpool University in 1979, and obtaining Fellow of the Royal College of Physicians in 1996. He was elected a Fellow of the Academy of Medical Sciences in 2009. He attended the Diploma in Tropical Medicine and Hygiene course at Liverpool School of Tropical Medicine in 1985 where he was awarded the Blacklock Medal for Parasitology and Entomology. Whitworth specializes in infectious diseases, epidemiology, and public health. Previous roles include working in The Gambia for Save the Children Fund on providing primary and secondary health care for Upper River Division. Subsequently he led investigations into ivermectin for onchocerciasis in Sierra Leone for the Medical Research Council, work for which he was awarded an M.D. with distinction in 1993. He was Team Leader for the Medical Research Council Programme on AIDS, based at the Uganda Virus Research Institute in Entebbe, from 1995 until 2002. When not living and working in Africa, Whitworth has been an academic staff member, specializing in HIV and vector-borne parasitic diseases, at both the Liverpool School of Tropical Medicine and the London School of Hygiene and Tropical Medicine.

Geoff Wong is Senior Lecturer in Primary Care at Queen Mary, University of London in the United Kingdom. He is an internationally and nationally recognised expert in realist review and evaluation. He has extensive expertise in undertaking and providing methodological support for both methods as well as in their methodological development. He recently completed a UK National Institute of Health Research funded project to develop quality and reporting standards and training materials for realist reviews (www.ramesesproject.org). He works part time as a Family Physician in the UK's National Health Service in London.

IOM STAFF

Charlee Alexander is a Senior Program Assistant with the IOM's Board on Global Health. Alexander graduated from the University of Chicago in 2010 with a B.A. in political science. After moving to Washington, DC, in September 2010, she worked as a legal assistant for the environmental firm Hill & Kehne, LLC, with a focus on brownfield remediation. Through the efforts of the RACER Trust, Alexander helped to revitalize and repurpose contaminated industrial properties remaining from the General Motors bankruptcy in 2009. Prior to joining the IOM, Charlee was a legal assistant at the civil rights firm Sanford Heisler, LLP, where the majority of her cases involved race and gender discrimination in the workplace. In October 2012, she traveled to Ghana for a 5-week child labor and trafficking volunteer program with a local NGO, the Cheerful Hearts Foundation. She conducted interviews with victims of child labor and their families to develop a socioeconomic snapshot of fishing communities. While Alexander has always been interested in civil and human rights, it was her trip to Ghana that gave her a public health focus.

Bridget Kelly is a Senior Program Officer with the IOM's Board on Global Health and the IOM/NRC Board on Children, Youth, and Families. She is the project co-director for the Workshop on Evaluation Methods for Large-Scale, Complex, Multi-National Global Health Initiatives and is also currently the study director for the Committee on the Science of Children Birth to Age 8: Deepening and Broadening the Foundation for Success. She also works on the DC Regional Public Health Case Challenge. Most recently she was the study co-director for the *Evaluation of PEPFAR*, an evaluation of U.S. global HIV/AIDS programs. Previously she was the study director for the report *Promoting Cardiovascular Health in the Developing World: A Critical Challenge to Achieve Global Health*, and she continues to direct a series of related follow-up activities on global chronic diseases, including the workshop Country-Level Decision Making for Control of Chronic Diseases. Her prior work has encompassed prevention of mental, emotional, and behavioral disorders; depression and parenting; and methodology for benefit-cost analysis. She was a 2007 Christine Mirzayan Science and Technology Policy Graduate Fellow at the National Academies. She holds an M.D. and a Ph.D. in neurobiology, both from Duke University, and a B.A. from Williams College, where she was also the recipient of the Hubbard Hutchinson Fellowship in fine arts. In addition to her background in science and health, she is a dancer and choreographer and has more than 10 years of experience in grassroots arts administration and production.

Kate Meck is an Associate Program Officer at the IOM. She is working on the African Tobacco Control project and the Evaluation Methods Workshop with the Board on Global Health, as well as a study to determine Diagnostic Criteria for ME/CFS with the Board on the Health of Select Populations. She previously worked on the *Evaluation of PEPFAR* and with the Committee on the U.S. Commitment to Global Health, the sequel to *America's Vital Interest in Global Health* (1997). Meck received her B.A. in international relations from American University, and her M.P.H. in global health program design, monitoring, and evaluation from GWU School of Public Health and Health Services.

Kimberly A. Scott has been a Senior Program Officer on the IOM's Board on Global Health since September 2005. She currently directs two forums: one on Global Violence Prevention and the other on Public Private Partnerships for Global Health and Safety. She is also co-directing a workshop on Evaluation Methods for Large-Scale, Complex, Multi-National Global Health Initiatives. From 2009 to 2013, she was the study co-director for the outcome and impact evaluation of the U.S. global HIV/AIDS initiative known as PEPFAR. Her portfolio of work for the IOM also includes a mix of consensus studies, workshops, and other activities: the Evaluation of the Implementation of the President's Emergency Plan for AIDS Relief (PEPFAR); Preventing Violence in Low- and Middle-Income Countries; the Assessment of the Role of Intermittent Preventive Treatment for Malaria in Infants; Depression, Parenting Practices, and the Health Development of Children; and Achieving Global Sustainable Surveillance for Zoonotic

Diseases. Prior to the IOM, she was an analyst on the health care team at the U.S. Government Accountability Office. Before returning to graduate school, she coordinated a foundation-funded program at Duke University's Center for Health Policy, Law, and Management to integrate public and private mental health services into the continuum of care for people living with and affected by HIV/AIDS in 54 counties in North Carolina. For 6 years, she served as the Executive Director of a Ryan White–funded HIV/AIDS consortium, developing a comprehensive ambulatory care system for 21 mostly rural counties in North Carolina. Previous North Carolina health-related committee service includes a number of advisory committees to the Governor of North Carolina and to the Secretary of North Carolina DHHS for programmatic and policy issues related to HIV care, prevention, and treatment, as well as substance abuse prevention and treatment. She received an M.S.P.H. in health policy analysis, from the University of North Carolina, Chapel Hill. As an Echols Scholar, she completed her undergraduate studies at the University of Virginia.

Appendix D

Evaluation Information Summary
for Core Example Initiatives

SCOPE OF THE EVALUATION

	PEPFAR	Global Fund	AMFm	PMI
Overarching evaluation aim/ question *What did the requestor and the evaluand want to know from the evaluation?*	Assess the performance and impact on health of PEPFAR-supported programs in partner countries and make recommendations for improvements	Assess the organizational efficiency and effectiveness of the Global Fund; the effectiveness of its partner environment; and the effects of increased resources on the reduction in the burden of the three diseases Study Area 1: Does the Global Fund, through both its policies and operations, reflect its critical core principles, including acting as a financial instrument (rather than as an implementation agency) and furthering country ownership; and in fulfilling these principles, whether it performs in an efficient and effective manner? Study Area 2: How effective and efficient is the Global Fund's partnership system in supporting HIV, tuberculosis (TB), and malaria programs at the country and global level? What are the wider effects of the Global Fund partnership on country systems?	To determine whether, and to what extent, AMFm Phase 1 achieves its objectives of (i) increasing availability of quality-assured ACTs (QAACTs) in outlets across the public, private for-profit, and not-for-profit sectors; (ii) increasing affordability of QAACTs to patients; (iii) increasing market share of QAACTs; and (iv) increasing use of QAACTs by patients, including vulnerable groups	Assess and evaluate the PMI program: Identify lessons learned across countries; assess population-based outcomes and impact; identify lessons and share experiences with other U.S. Government (USG) engagements in global health initiatives

		Study Area 3: What is the impact of scaling up against HIV, TB, and malaria? What is the Global Fund's contribution?		
Requestor of the evaluation *Who asked for the evaluation?*	U.S. Congress (mandated in PEPFAR reauthorization legislation)	Global Fund Board	Global Fund Board	PMI Leadership
Funder of the evaluation *Who paid for the evaluation?*	U.S. Department of State, Office of the U.S. Global AIDS Coordinator (OGAC)	Global Fund	Global Fund	USAID through contractor GH Tech
Primary intended audiences *(For whom is the evaluation primarily performed based on the statement of task or terms of reference or the intent communicated by the requestor/funder?)*	U.S. Congress OGAC PEPFAR implementers (USG agencies, country programs, implementing partners)	Global Fund	The Global Fund Board, to guide its decision on whether to "expand, accelerate, modify, terminate, or suspend the AMFm business line"	PMI, USAID, CDC

SCOPE OF THE EVALUATION

	PEPFAR	Global Fund	AMFm	PMI
Secondary audiences *Other major audiences for the evaluation findings*	PEPFAR partner country stakeholders (government and nongovernment) Global HIV stakeholders (e.g., multilateral agencies, other bilateral and foundation donors, advocates)	Global Fund funders Global Fund partner countries Global HIV stakeholders (e.g., other multilateral agencies, bilateral and foundation donors, advocates)	AMFm pilot country malaria program managers, global malaria stakeholders (bilateral and multilateral agencies, Roll Back Malaria, etc.).	U.S. Congress, other USG global health implementers PMI countries both national program personnel and USG personnel
Time period of the evaluated initiative that was assessed in the evaluation	2003–2012	After one complete (5-year) grant cycle 2002–2007, data collection through 2009	2010–2011. The period started from the point of signature of AMFm country grants (mid-2010 onward to the completion of data collection. Endline outlet surveys were completed in December 2011; data collection for additional studies (remote areas and logo studies) was completed in April 2012; household survey data from 2011 to July 12 were included.	2005–2010
Total budget of evaluated initiative during	$28.5 billion (current USD) appropriated to PEPFAR country	$4.96 billion (2002–2007) $9.97 billion (2002–2009)	$216 million copayment fund (to Feb 2012) + $42.4 million for	$1.2 billion for the first 5 years of the PMI project (FY2006–FY2010)

the time period covered in the evaluation			supporting interventions (disbursed to Nov 2011)	programs from FY2004–FY2011 (see Figure 4-3, p. 103, IOM's 2013 *Evaluation of PEPFAR* report)
Duration of the evaluation	2009–2013 (45 months, separated into planning and implementation phases	2007–2009 (23 months)	April 2009 to December 2012	May–November 2011
Cost of the evaluation	$8.2 million USD	Almost $17 million USD for the three distinct evaluations	$10.7 million USD	$292,935 USD [Boston University [BU] Purchase Order only) Three additional consultant members of the Evaluation Team were paid directly by GH Tech outside of the BU contract
Geographic scope of the evaluation *How many countries/regions were included in the scope of the evaluation?*	"Whole of PEPFAR": Scope varied by data source, ranging from all countries receiving PEPFAR funds (100+ countries) to the subset of countries where most investment was focused (31 countries submitting country operational plans at time of evaluation) to a subset of those countries with in-depth data collected (13 countries)	Whole of Global Fund; scope with regard to data collection varied by study area; 16 countries for SA 2 and 18 countries for SA 3	All 8 Phase 1 pilot countries (Ghana, Kenya, Madagascar, Niger, Nigeria, Tanzania (mainland), Uganda, Zanzibar)	15 PMI focus countries in Africa

GOVERNANCE STRUCTURE AND REPORT

	PEPFAR	Global Fund	AMFm	PMI
Evaluators: Structure and composition of evaluation team, subteams, subcontractors, and advisory mechanisms	Single IOM evaluation team composed of a committee of volunteer experts; the IOM staff; and paid consultants for both qualitative and quantitative methods Evaluation team was divided into subteams for data collection field visits and into working groups by topic area An external panel of expert volunteers reviewed the evaluation report prior to release to the evaluand and the public	Independent consultants conducted three interlinked studies Macro International was awarded the contract for the evaluation of all three areas and enlisted a consortium of different universities and service providers, including Johns Hopkins University, Harvard School of Public Health, Washington University, Axios International, Development Finance International (DFI), the Indian Institute for Health Management Research, the African Population and Health Research Centre, and WHO	ICF international was the primary contractor for the independent evaluation (IE), with a subcontract to the London School of Hygiene and Tropical Medicine Outlet survey data collection was contracted separately by the Global Fund, without a direct line of accountability between the data collectors and the IE The AMFm Ad Hoc Committee provided oversight of the evaluation and reported the findings to the Board. The TERG provided guidance on the technical parameters of the evaluation design; an Expert Advisory Group advised the Global Fund secretariat	The evaluation was managed by Management Firm (GH Tech), which subcontracted the evaluation to BU and three independent consultants The evaluation team (made up of the BU team and the three consultants) consisted of members with broad public health experience, malaria expertise, extensive experience in the use of both quantitative and qualitative methods, and proven experience in complex multicountry evaluations Evaluation team was divided into groups to visit different countries and address the different evaluation objectives

Relationship of evaluator to evaluand *For example: Independent external contractor; internal independent evaluation unit within the same organization as the evaluand; internally conducted by evaluand*	Independent and external	Independent and external	Independent and external	Independent and external

GOVERNANCE STRUCTURE AND REPORT

	PEPFAR	Global Fund	AMFm	PMI
Oversight mechanisms *For example, legislative oversight, oversight mechanisms in the evaluator's institution, oversight by the evaluand or the evaluand's advisory bodies*	Oversight by the IOM standard mechanisms governing consensus studies, including committee formation processes to ensure balance and avoid conflicts of interest; compliance with transparency requirements of the Federal Advisory Committee Act; external report review OGAC appointed a liaison, the head of Strategic Information, to whom the IOM staff could communicate their needs for evaluation (i.e., data and documentation requests, interview scheduling; information needed for the IOM logistics planning for field work, etc.)	Oversight of the evaluation was provided by the TERG. The TERG is an advisory body that provides independent assessment and advice to the Global Fund Board and advises the Global Fund Secretariat. The TERG organized regular consultative meetings with the contractor to assess progress and discuss issues	Building on prior work completed by the Roll Back Malaria Partnership, the Global Fund Secretariat, with input from the TERG, AMFm Ad Hoc Committee, AMFm Phase 1 country officials, Expert Advisory Group, and key technical partners, prepared the initial evaluation design which was put out to tender AMFm Ad Hoc Committee met approximately twice per year and received process updates and interim evaluation findings (e.g., baseline results) On encouragement of the Independent Evaluation (IE) team and TERG, the Ad Hoc Committee, with TERG Chair,	GH Tech had administrative oversight The Evaluation Team submitted a draft report for comments to the PMI, USAID, and CDC staff members. The Evaluation Team reviewed the comments and responded, as they deemed appropriate

				identified independent consultants to propose "success benchmarks"
Reporting requirements *Frequency of reports, such as preliminary, periodic, final reports*	Two reports were published during the evaluation period: (1) Planning report after the planning phase (1.5 years) that detailed the strategic approach to the evaluation and evaluability assessments but no preliminary findings (2) Final report with findings, conclusions, and recommendations at the conclusion of the evaluation	A number of interim reports were submitted to the TERG for review Final reports were released by the independent consultants for each of the three study areas A synthesis report, based on findings and recommendations of the final study area reports, was also released by Marco International	Three reports were published: Inception report, baseline report and final report. In addition, a supplement with the results of the secondary analysis of household data on antimalarial use was published separately from the main report because data became available after the main report was completed	Periodic and draft reports were submitted to the management firm for transmission to evaluand. Comments and feedback were incorporated into the final report as appropriate. The Evaluation Team had full discretion to accept or reject comments as they saw fit
Evaluand's access to preliminary findings or draft reports	Per institutional requirements of the IOM, the evaluand had no access to preliminary findings or draft reports before final release	Preliminary and progress reports were submitted regularly to the TERG, and were discussed in detail with the contractor	The evaluand had the opportunity to comment on reports before they were finalized	The PMI had access to the draft report; they shared it with personnel from USAID and CDC

GOVERNANCE STRUCTURE AND REPORT

	PEPFAR	Global Fund	AMFm	PMI
Authorship and ownership of evaluation findings/report	Final report authored by the convened committee and issued by the IOM; content of the report belongs to the IOM	Final reports for each of the three study areas, as well as a synthesis report, were authored by the independent contractors and released by Marco International The TERG released a summary for the synthesis report and each of the three study areas In the summaries for each study area, the TERG provided an "assessment" of and comments on each of the contractor's recommendations	All reports authored by the IE team; the content of the report belongs to the IE team	Final report authored by the Evaluation Team; content of the report belongs to the Evaluation Team
Other notable aspects of the Terms of Reference *Any other issues not mentioned above*	Congressional mandate for study afforded limited ability to negotiate terms, which lead to necessity of communication/ explanation to clarify appropriate expectations with respect to complying with specific terms of the mandate	The TERG emphasized that the contractor should ensure a clear focus on capacity building in the conduct of evaluations under SA 3, not necessarily building or strengthening systems, but that dormant capacity at the country level should be mobilized by the contractor and in-country Impact Evaluation Task Force	While the original terms of reference for the evaluation called for household surveys to measure antimalarial use, these were not included in the final evaluation design because of budget implications. Instead, data from national surveys that were	None noted

appropriately timed (close to baseline and endline) were to be used to report on use. In the end, these were only available for five of the pilots, which did not include the two "fastest-moving" pilots, Ghana and Kenya

EVALUATION APPROACH

	PEPFAR	Global Fund	AMFm	PMI
Evaluability assessments *What assessments were conducted before the evaluation was conducted? For example, exploration of program's objectives, activities, and theory of change; data mapping, assessment of available/accessible data; assessment of feasibility of data collection; evaluation design development, including analysis of methodological issues; and assessment of how evaluation findings can improve the*	Two-year design and operational planning phase prior to the evaluation implementation phase included • Clarification and interpretation of the evaluation mandate • Research on PEPFAR's legislative and programmatic intent and objectives, program design, complexity, and operational structure • Design planning to choose conceptual framework; methods to be applied and analytical plan; develop in-depth evaluation questions; map data availability, accessibility, and quality Evaluability assessments continued and	The TERG nominated an Impact Evaluation Task Force in each of the countries that were to participate The TERG developed the scope of work, study design, and research questions for the evaluation, and upon approval by the Global Fund Board, identified the independent consultant to carry out evaluation activities, after a competitive bidding process	An AMFm Phase 1 Monitoring and Evaluation Technical Framework was developed by the Global Fund Secretariat with input from a broad range of stakeholders, including the TERG, AMFm Ad Hoc Committee, AMFm Phase 1 country officials and technical partners, which included elements of the proposed independent evaluation and data mapping for national level surveys planned to be implemented by others The data collection and analysis methods for the outlet surveys that had been developed by the ACTwatch project were adapted for use in the IE	On an annual basis, the PMI team compiles all routine data, together with any survey data or data from other nonroutine sources (resistance monitoring, special studies, etc.) into an annual report. This report provides a summary of the various data collected during the year, examines progress and trends, and points out areas for improvements or enhancements in the coming year

	adjustments were made during the implementation phase as needed			
program or its objectives *For example, quasi-experimental; theory of change; case study*				
Overall evaluation approach	Retrospective, quasi-cross-sectional, time trend, nonexperimental, mixed methods approach using program impact pathway logic model framework; hybrid case-study approach by country and by topic area; benchmarking analysis for legislative, policy, and other programmatic objectives	Retrospective, nonexperimental, mixed methods; separate examination of different study areas; country case studies employing interviews with stakeholders, program managers, and Global Fund staff as well as household and facility surveys and health information system record reviews in the areas of HIV/AIDS, TB, and malaria	Nonexperimental design with a pre-test and post-test assessment, with each country treated independently as a case study. Nationally representative outlet surveys conducted at baseline and endline. Assessment of context and process factors using key informants and document review. Theory of change used to interpret and attribute changes, based on logic model together with context and process factors. Additional studies conducted outlet surveys to explore QAACT price, availability, and market share in remote areas of two countries (Ghana and Kenya) and qualitative methods to study understanding of the AMFm logo (in four countries)	Mixed methods approach using document review, key-informant interviews, field visits, electronic surveys, and trend analysis of publically available and relevant datasets

EVALUATION APPROACH

	PEPFAR	Global Fund	AMFm	PMI
Sampling used *How were choices made about the program components to evaluate? How was sampling done for data collection/analysis?*	Program areas evaluated were determined by mapping closely to the Statement of Task and the initiative's predetermined technical areas Comprehensive sample for most financial data (all PEPFAR countries) Existing sample for program monitoring data (PEPFAR's preexisting selection of countries writing country operational plans) Existing sample for clinical data (PEPFAR's preexisting selection of Track 1.0 implementing partners)	**Program Components:** Priority evaluation questions for the Five Year Evaluation were discussed, reviewed and refined by the TERG; input was sought from the Board of the Global Fund and through an extensive stakeholder consultation **Sampling for data collection/analysis:** Purposive sampling of countries for evaluation of impact (SA 3) (n=20) and for SA 2 (n=16) considering the following criteria: 1. Regional and disease balance 2. Availability of existing impact and baseline data 3. Magnitude of Global Fund disbursement 4. Duration of programming 5. Opportunities for partner harmonization	Outlet survey sample sizes estimated for each country to be able to detect a 20 percentage point change between baseline and endline in QAACT availability, separately for rural and urban domains, pooling across outlet types and sectors. The ACTwatch cluster sampling approach was used. A full census was undertaken in Zanzibar. Key informants were selected purposefully	Core objectives were evaluated based on the PMI evaluation framework: Leadership, Management, and Resources (Obj 1); Putting Core Operating Principles into Practice (Obj 2); Wider Partnership Environment (Obj 3); Assess Program Outcomes and Impacts (Obj 4); Assess Operational Research Activities (Obj 5); and Make Actionable Recommendations (Obj 6) Purposeful sampling for key informant; Systematic literature reviews for document review. Countries for field visit selected by evaluand based on countries with at least two malaria survey (Malaria Indicator Survey or DHS) data points

| Data types/Data sources | Purposeful sampling for in-depth qualitative data collection (interviews and some document review)

Systematic literature reviews for some document review | Financial data
Routine program monitoring data
Program clinical data
Semi-structured interview data
Document review
Globally reported indicator data | **Study Area 1:** interviews, an organizational development (OD) assessment of Global Fund governance and management, performance review, benchmarking of results and processes, and document review

Study Area 2: In-depth qualitative assessments (850 interviews), extensive literature review and in-depth review and analysis of performance data on Global Fund grants

Study Area 3: National health accounts, district facility censuses, household surveys, civil society organization surveys, record reviews, and follow-up studies of patients | Outlet surveys
Key informant interviews and document review
Focus group discussions
Secondary analysis of household survey data | Routine program monitoring data
Semi-structured interview data
Document review
Globally reported malaria data |

EVALUATION APPROACH

	PEPFAR	Global Fund	AMFm	PMI
Data analysis methods and triangulation for mixed methods	Analysis and interpretation within each data type appropriate to methodological standards Iterative interpretation and triangulation within and across data types, sources, and investigators	Study Area 3: The evaluation study design used a stepwise approach to examine trends in health outcomes, coverage, and risk behaviors; access and quality of services; and funding Secondary analysis of existing data and record reviews were conducted in 18 countries, and new data collection was carried out in 8 of these countries	Analysis used a predetermined tabulation plan, and adjusted for the survey design A theory of change developed for AMFm was used to integrate findings across outlet surveys and context/process documentation	Iterative interpretation and triangulation within and across data types, sources, and investigators

DISSEMINATION AND UPTAKE OF EVALUATION FINDINGS, CONCLUSIONS, AND RECOMMENDATIONS

	PEPFAR	Global Fund	AMFm	PMI
Report materials and other communications products beyond the required reports	Report summary (15 pages) Report Summary booklet with chapter main messages (~100 pages) Report brief (4 pages) Online interactive experiences	Summaries of each study area Each country participating in the impact study (SA 3) produced its own evaluation report (n=18)	Main report (403 pages) and appendixes (287 pages), which includes a short summary (5 pages) and a longer executive summary (45 pages) Supplementary report on antimalarial use, based on household survey data (68 pages)	N/A

			Lancet paper (Tougher et al.), published November 2012	
Dissemination activities	Briefings with congressional staff; OGAC; USG agencies	Local presentation of results of the country-level impact evaluation, particularly household and facility survey and record review results	Feedback to country programs (June 2012); presentations to AMFm ad hoc committee, the AMFm Working Group, and the MDAG (July–October 2012) in lead up to board meeting November 2012	Briefings with congressional staff (public event co-hosted by PATH) and USG agencies
	Public briefing events (all webcast)	Summary reports by the Global Fund, posting of reports on the Global Fund website		Online dissemination of final report
	Presentations at conferences and meetings	The TERG briefings of the Global Fund Board	Presentations at International Health Economics Association, American Society of Tropical Medicine and Hygiene (ASTMH), Multilateral Initiative on Malaria (MIM), DFID	
	Published commentaries			

DISSEMINATION AND UPTAKE OF EVALUATION FINDINGS, CONCLUSIONS, AND RECOMMENDATIONS

	PEPFAR	Global Fund	AMFm	PMI
Responses to evaluation	PEPFAR did an internal written response to the recommendations Bidirectional exchange between the IOM and implementing agencies during technical briefings about specific considerations for recommendations and agency implementation Commentaries in journals and blog postings authored by stakeholders external to the IOM	The TERG summaries of final study area reports Global Fund Secretariat implemented provisions to address some observations and recommendations	Written feedback received from the TERG and from the AMFm Working Group Commentaries in scientific journals and media coverage	The PMI generated a management report identifying which recommendations they wished to act upon and describing how they would implement the proposed changes The report was highlighted on the PMI website and broadly disseminated electronically
Mechanisms for tracking implementation of recommendations or impact of the evaluation	The IOM has limited formal and resourced internal mechanisms for tracking recommendation implementation and other report impact	Unknown	No formal mechanism for tracking impact of the evaluation	Beyond the scope of the Evaluation Team

OTHER

	PEPFAR	Global Fund	AMFm	PMI
What other information should be known that influenced or informed the evaluation?	Not a financial audit or an evaluation of the operational structure of PEPFAR or its placement within the USG Not an evaluation of the U.S. contribution to the Global Fund or of programming and funding to NIH Committee interpreted additional areas of study not explicitly stated in mandate but determined to be needed to be responsive to the charge (i.e., funding, knowledge management, country ownership, and sustainability)	There was early realization that it would be impossible to separate the potential impacts of the different funding/donor mechanisms on disease burden	Implementation period was short: 6.5–15.5 months from first arrival of copaid drugs; some countries had not commenced supporting interventions at the time of endline data collection Preliminary findings presented to consultative forum of country stakeholders for review and debate	Evaluation Team was asked to avoid comparing the PEPFAR mechanisms with the PMI approach Evaluation Team had very little country-level financial data Evaluation Team was constrained by lack of multiple time data points to assess country trends and impacts

SOURCE: Information compiled from evaluation summary documents and members of the respective evaluation teams.

Appendix E

Evaluation Design Resources Highlighted at the Workshop

Resource	Description	Source
The International Initiative for Impact Evaluation (3ie)	3ie's mission as an international organization is to increase development effectiveness through better use of evidence in developing countries	http://www.3ieimpact.org
BetterEvaluation Rainbow Framework Planning Tool	A planning tool used to plan, commission, manage, and check the quality of an evaluation	http://betterevaluation.org
"Broadening the range of designs and methods for impact evaluations"	A summary report of a study on impact evaluation commissioned by the Department for International Development in the United Kingdom	Stern, E., N. Stame, J. Mayne, K. Forss, R. Davies, and B. Befani. 2012. http://r4d.dfid.gov.uk/pdf/outputs/misc_infocomm/DFIDWorkingPaper38.pdf
"Addressing attribution of cause and effect in small n impact evaluations: Toward an integrated framework"	A working paper by Howard White and Daniel Phillips of 3ie examining approaches for small-scale evaluation	White, H., and D. Phillips. 2012. http://www.3ieimpact.org/media/filer/2012/06/29/working_paper_15.pdf